The Core Strength Workout

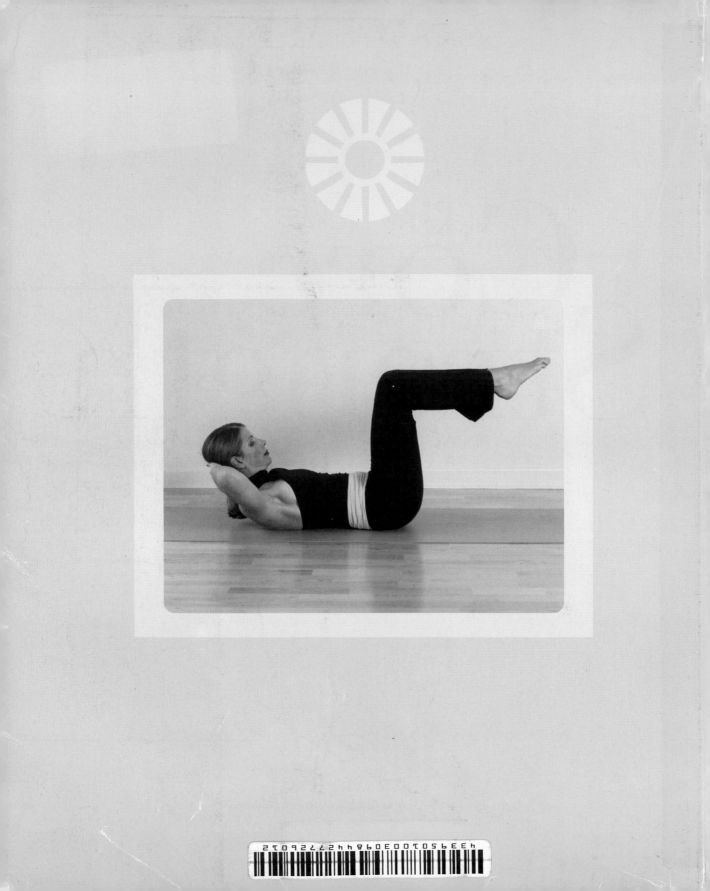

Karon Karter

The Core Strength Workout

Get Flat Abs and a Healthy Back

Pilates • Yoga • Exercise Ball

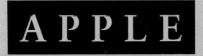

Text © 2004 by Karon Karter
Photographs © 2003 by Fair Winds Press

Published in the UK in 2004 by
Apple Press
Sheridan House
112-116A Western Road
Hove
East Sussex BN3 1DD
England

10 9 8 7 6 5 4 3 2 1

ISBN 1-84092-454-3

Cover design by Mary Ann Smith
Book layout and production by Laura Herrmann Design
Photography by Bobbie Bush Photography, www.bobbiebush.com

Printed and bound in Singapore

*The information in this book is for educational purposes only. It is not intended to replace
the advice of a physician or medical practitioner. Please see your health care provider
before beginning any new health program.*

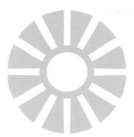

TO MY MOTHER, FOR BEING MY BEST FRIEND

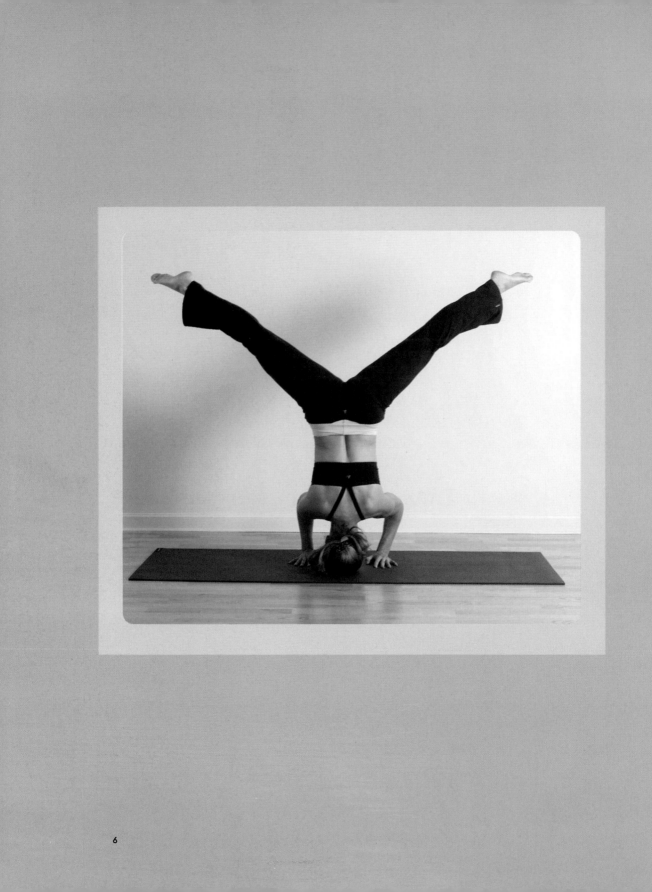

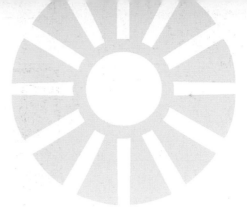

contents

FOREWORD

I have a fun life. As the Director for the Center of Human Performance and Nutrition Research at The Cooper Institute, I pretty much get to see it all. I get to work with elite athletes, including one of Europe's premier professional cycling teams, as well as people who are severely unfit. While the pro cyclists will generate power outputs of 500 or more watts during an exercise, the latter population will do well to break 110. In the middle of those two extremes is everyone else!

However, if you are an exercise physiology sort of guy, this is a great place to work. I have the opportunity to work with, in, and around a variety of populations with the specific aim of improving health, freedom from disease, and human performance through exercise. It does not matter who you are—exercise benefits everyone.

While this may seem like a pretty lofty statement, consider the facts: Time and time again, exercise has consistently been shown to decrease the incidence of diseases such as cancer, diabetes, heart disease, arthritis and a variety of others. Every year the list gets longer and longer. In essence, physical activity performed on a consistent basis gives you life. Despite all the benefits associated with regular exercise, it is still sad to see that only twenty-five percent of our population exercises on a regular basis.

This is difficult for me to figure out as exercise gives us most of the things that we want out of life pertaining to health. These include a reduction in disease, a decreased risk for mortality, an improvement in everything related to cardiovascular health, a better sense of well-being, and many of the "freedoms" found from being able to move and go about our daily tasks more easily. The concept and practice of maintaining core stability is essential to all of these benefits.

In a very literal sense, core stability is exactly what it sounds like—those aspects of health that lie at the heart, center, and groundwork of our muscle and skeletal system. Our core forms the foundation from which we impart movement every day of our lives. From the moment we rise in the morning, to the moment we lay ourselves down to sleep, our core musculature plays a role in getting us through the day more easily and more safely.

Need an example? Okay, have you ever bruised a rib or hurt your lower back? Most of us have. Have you ever noticed that when this happens almost every movement you make causes discomfort? Standing, sitting, coughing, sneezing, turning to take your groceries out of the car! The list goes on and on. The reason is fairly simple. It is because those areas of your body are part of your core or foundational system that stabilize and refine the small movements necessary to protect your back and maintain your posture. When you damage them, every movement is affected.

The good news is that is does not take a lot of time or a lot of effort to improve your core strength. Better yet, you can do the exercises at home, in a group, in a hotel room—almost anywhere. All it takes is a little practice and a little guidance to set you on your way. That is the beauty of Karon Karter's *Core Strength Workout*.

Core strength has been around for centuries and in many forms. Yoga always comes to mind as one of the original forms, as does Pilates. It is this latter form of core stability exercises that Karon highlights in this easy-to-use book, designed specifically to help you improve your core strength.

I have had the privilege knowing Karon for many years. We worked together in the same fitness center while I was doing my doctoral studies and she has been a champion of health promotion for as long as I have known her. One of the things I have found is that Karon is someone who is genuinely concerned with promoting the health of the individual, rather than jumping on the popular bandwagons promoting "cosmetic health." You know the type: Do a zillion crunches per day, eat like a cricket and make sure that you are tan and seen in the popular and trendy classes of the day. Karon's approach has always been different.

Targeting the individual, Karon brings a refreshing approach to functional fitness and the practice of core stability training. Better yet, with Karon you get the results of the trendy classes and come out the other side of your program fit, more stable, and looking and feeling better. She has a real life approach to real life solutions that help you meet real life goals. In this book, Karon exemplifies her teaching ability by giving you a series of exercises that are beneficial and functional.

Enjoy *The Core Strength Workout*. It has something for everyone, which is the ultimate goal of fitness in the first place. Whether you are out of shape or on the opposite extreme of the fitness spectrum, *The Core Strength Workout* has something for you.

Conrad Earnest, PhD, FACSM
Director, Center for Human Performance & Nutrition Research
The Cooper Institute Centers for Integrated Health Research

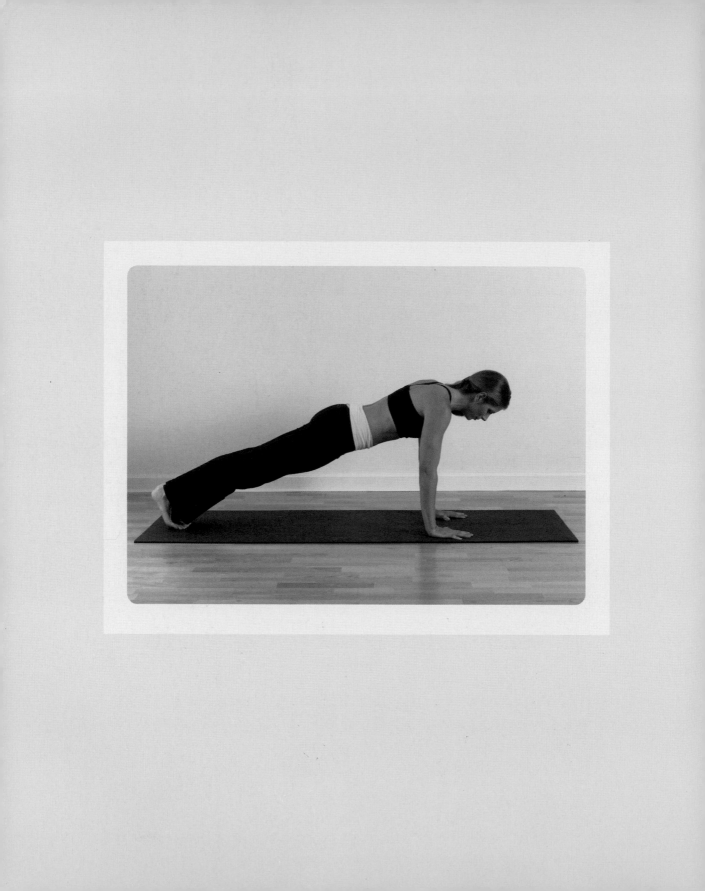

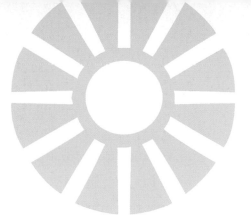

Introduction

My core strength journey began just about seven years ago after I took my first Pilates class. I'll never forget the feeling—I loved it despite rolling and flopping all over the mat. I clearly remember thinking, "I need more of this in my body." After many years of fitness—I had interned and worked for the Cooper Institute for Aerobics Research, survived teaching aerobics class in New York City, and had put endless mileage on my car by teaching fitness in just about every club in Dallas—I couldn't do a Teaser, which is a Pilates exercise that tests your core strength. As I have since learned, the core initiates most movement in your body. It extends from the base of your neck to the muscles between your legs and is made up of overlapping layers of muscles, consisting of all the muscles in your abdomen, back, hips and pelvic floors. When I found out how weak my core was, I knew something was missing in my workout. Fitness came easy; Pilates did not! I clearly remember my master instructor, Colleen Glenn, saying, "You can't learn Pilates in a weekend." She was so right!

By the time I had completed my Pilates certification, I had put in hundreds of hours, which included lots of classes, private sessions, an eight week pre-certification course along with four grueling months of weekend workshops. All in all, three years! But, I had core strength and body awareness—probably the best two gifts that I could give myself. I could walk into any yoga class or attend a stability ball workshop with confidence, knowing my body and its limitations. These are my goals for you! Whether traveling from yoga to Pilates classes or working out in the privacy of your own living room, I hope you attain a certain amount of body awareness and core strength so that you move toward your best body.

Of course while I'm passionate about Pilates, it's just one avenue to core strength. Yoga is another, and stability balls are rolling out as the next "it" workout, which is why *The Core Strength Workout* provides the best of those workouts so you can develop real core strength—and enhance your life!

Your journey begins in Chapter One, "Centering Your Workout," in which you'll learn what core strength is and how it can change your life. Amazing abs and a fitter figure are obvious benefits, but, core strength also enhances your sex life! Interested yet? In that case, Chapter Two, "Invisible Lift," gets you started. I firmly believe that you need a starting place, and evaluating your own posture is it. I can also promise you that good posture is just the beginning of body confidence and beating the back blues. Did you know that lower back pain sends more people throbbing to the doctor than a headache? You don't have to be a statistic. By strengthening your core, you can provide a first layer of defense against back pain. Chapter Three, "Core Concepts," is about body awareness and helps you to discover that being able to live comfortably in your own skin is about self-discovery. Being truthful about what's happening in your body right now is how you can change the things you can and accept the things you can't change. This chapter, then, provides the fundamentals for the exercises to come. These core concepts will help you do the exercises correctly and safely. Only then are you ready for the workouts. Chapter Four, "Wake up Your Core," is the next best thing to a private lesson with step-by-by instructions for beginners. This chapter will deepen and intensify your knowledge of core strength and will start your journey to heightened body awareness as you learn basic exercises that teach you how to tap into your breath and body.

As you advance, Chapter Five, "Core Curves," deepens your core connection. This is the intermediate workout, which begins to focus on muscles other than your core, such as your inner thigh and pelvic floor muscles. Strengthening these muscles—the same muscles that contract during an orgasm—also enhances your sex life! And finally, in Chapter Six, "Core Strength for Life," I provide advanced exercises to tighten and tone your body from head to toe; it's a total body workout that reshapes your body and trains your brain. Developing skill in movement while attaining total body strength is what this chapter is about.

Although you will see and feel changes in your body fairly quickly, you can do these exercises for a long time because they'll continue to deliver results, regardless of how long you practice them. As you gain in strength and flexibility, the exercises then challenge you to work so deeply in your own body that you physically feel your core contract. But this feeling takes time to develop, which is why these exercises get you to slow down and consciously think before moving your body. That's what makes this program a mind and body workout.

When you're ready to begin, here are a few pointers to help you get the most of this core strength program. First, pay attention to your body. If you have any lower back pain while doing these exercises, please see a doctor. It is a good idea to talk with your doctor before starting any fitness program, or you might also consider using this book under the guidance of a physical therapist or a well-respected physical trainer. Second, keep a journal of your workouts, so you can record how you feel. Changing your lifestyle, work, and exercise habits isn't easy. A journal can help determine how you're evolving toward your best body. Third, at times, we all need incentives to get moving. Find a reward system that works for you. I love fitness, but there are days when I don't want to work out. Knowing this, I will buy a new exercise outfit only if I accomplish my exercise goals for that week. It helps—and you have to make the decision to keep moving regardless of what life throws your way! And finally, set realistic goals. Spending two hours in the gym is not practical if you're juggling diaper changing and vegetable chopping. Yet, find time for yourself; otherwise, you won't be much use to your loved ones or anything else you pursue in life. Slow and steady gets your best body!

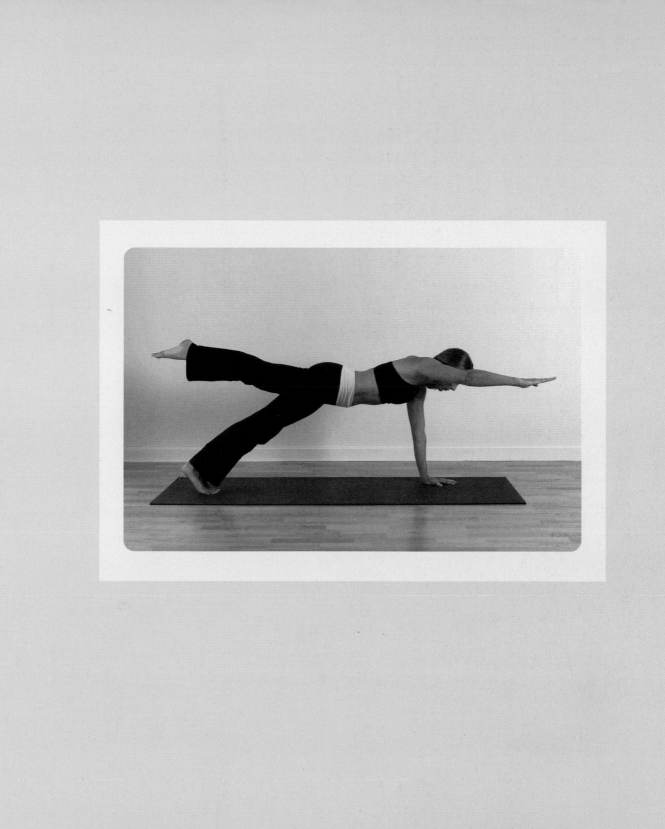

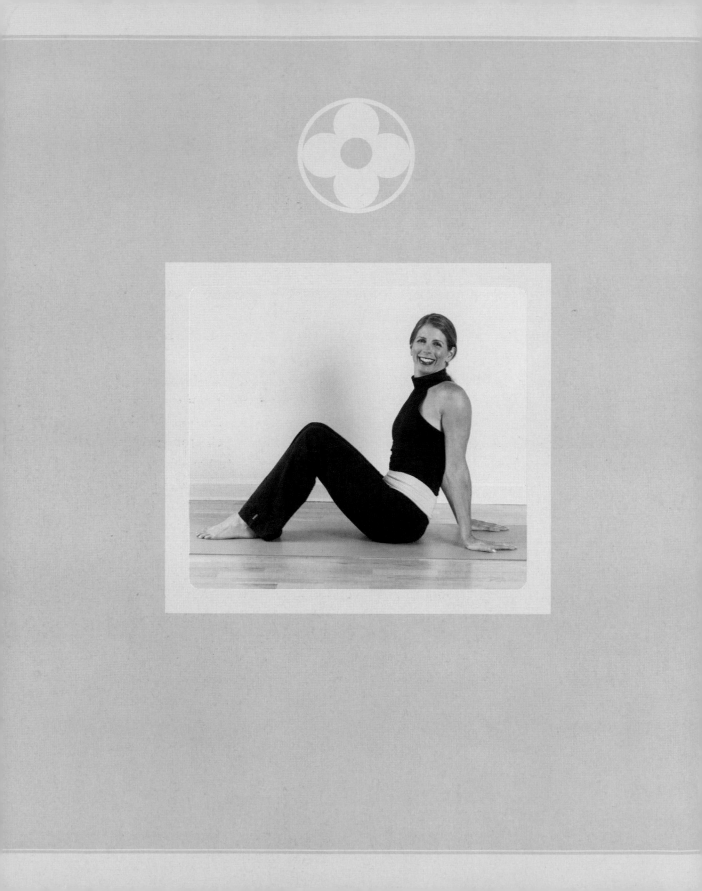

Chapter 1

Centering Your Workout

Sure, the exercises in this book tighten and trim your torso and super-slim your body—all great goals—but *The Core Strength Workout* will also change your life. This book does not focus on what you should not do; rather it concentrates on what you can do to feel more alive, and what you need to do to achieve the life you want. Optimal health does not just happen. It is built over time, beginning with small steps, not a sudden lifestyle change. The choices you make every day to create a balanced and healthy life will have an impact on your sense of wellness now—and in the future. Most importantly, good health is not equivalent to "just getting by" or not getting sick; it is living life with vitality and optimism, having enough energy to pursue your dreams and goals, and living life in a capable body. Core strength, then, is your express ticket to ultra-amazing abs, plus good health. Now is the perfect time to focus on core strength—what it is and how to get more of it—because *the stronger your core, the better your body works, looks, and feels!*

Your core initiates movement; it's made up of overlapping layers of muscles, extending from the base of your neck to the muscles between your legs and consists of all the muscles in your abdomen, back, and pelvic floors. Although these muscles play various roles in the body, they mostly provide support for your spine. If your core is weak, then you are more susceptible to injury. Core strength changes you physically as well as how you feel about your body.

A STRONG CORE:

- provides stability for your spine and its movements, such as rotation and extension of the spine

- stabilizes the muscles of your midsection, including the hips and pelvis, so movement, such as walking or running, is enhanced

- reduces the strain on the limbs because the core takes on more of the workload

- keeps injury-prone areas healthy by reducing overall strain; two classic examples are the over-worked lower back and delicate shoulder joints

- governs various joints in the body, so they maintain their position during movement

Imagine that your body is a chain with one link stacked on top of another to build a heavy-duty and hard-wearing chain. Any weak link can destroy the chain's integrity. Your body is built upon a carefully balanced system of muscle, ligament, tendon, fascia (connective tissue), and bone. Each group works interdependently, but they all depend on one another. Your body is only as strong as the muscles providing stability for your bones as well as the muscles moving them. If one set of muscles fail, then the pairing muscle group picks up the slack and, in the process, stresses the attached joint. Weak muscles, especially your core muscles, make your body more vulnerable to injury.

This is why *The Core Strength Workout* is so important. I strongly believe that your core is the weakest link in the body when, in fact, it should be the strongest. *Not only does your core support your spine, all movement begins with your core and its strength can provide a first necessary layer of defense against pain and injury.* But that's not all. Strengthening your core will also make all your movements a little easier and life in general a whole lot healthier.

During my fourteen years of studying, teaching, and writing about fitness, I have compiled the very extensive list of exercises that fills these pages. These exercises are for life. So, take your time with this book. Pick a workout that fits your exercise level and try to get through the entire sequence of exercises. Each workout combines a coordinated set of strengthening and stretching moves to balance and realign muscle groups that have either been neglected or not trained correctly in the first place. I will *not* ask you to give up your current exercise program—only to add these exercises at least two days a week to complement what you're already doing. At first, you might only notice a tighter, trimmer torso. But this book goes much further to guide you toward a smarter health plan integrating all levels of fitness to reshape your body and train your mind.

THE CORE STRENGTH WORKOUT WILL:

Strengthen your core: With these moves, the center of your body, which begins between your legs and extends to the base of your neck, will become strong, healthy, toned, and ready for any challenge!

Heighten the mind and body connection: You will connect your mind to your body and your body to your mind by asking them to work together so each move becomes thoughtful, rather than an afterthought. Body awareness is vital to permanent change; understanding your body—its flaws and all—makes this workout holistic in nature.

Improve your sense of balance: Most people take balance for granted. It is only when they age or suffer a fall that they realize balance plays a vital role in their daily lives. You will improve your balance skills with these core strength exercises, particularly when using the exercise ball.

Develop a balanced body: This integrated training approach strengthens the muscles of the body as a whole, using multiple muscle groups in each exercise, which helps reduce muscle imbalances and prepares your body for real life movements.

Diminish unwanted dimples: With these exercises, inches shrink and dimples disappear. You will tighten and trim your body, so you can feel ready to show off your firm and fabulous body in your favorite form-fitting jeans or that skimpy bikini!

Gain in range of motion: You can relieve stiffness and pain in your body by improving your range of motion through stretching. Restricted movements and lack of flexibility begin the downward spiral that can lead to an injury. Key exercises I present will extend and rotate the spine to keep it flexible and lengthened. The flexibility of your joints will also improve. Achieving optimal muscle flexibility will allow the joints to move smoothly through their normal range of motion. Short muscles feel tight and tense. Stretching releases tension and restores working muscles to their natural length so you can relax and move freely.

Find your breath: Every exercise presented here is coordinated with the breath to strengthen your core, purify your blood, relax your body, and increase your circulation. These exercises will also work to strengthen the muscles around your lungs and improve your breathing capacity.

Enhance your sex life: The core begins between your legs, in an area of muscles called the pelvic floors. By strengthening these muscles, which also contract during orgasm, you will enjoy deeper, more intense orgasms. You will also strengthen the muscles of the pelvis, so you may find that you have more control over your hips, and increased levels of stamina—features that will surely bring pleasure to you and your partner!

An Ancient Science with a New Twist

Core workouts are not a new concept. Just two decades ago, yoga seemed an ocean away, while today it is breathing a new life into every workout. And nothing works like Pilates when it comes to strengthening your core. Joseph Pilates (1880-1967) adapted and refined yoga and various other Greek and Roman exercise regimes to invent a hybrid series of exercises that strengthen the body, particularly the core, while elongating the muscles, which avoids the bulky weight room look. Despite core workouts extending back nearly 2000 years, core fitness is buzzing today. But why now? Perhaps it is the desire for that six-pack look, which, after all, we all want. But, more importantly, these workouts give you real core strength. My students have come to believe wholeheartedly in core strength. Over the years, I have shown hundreds of students that the secret to having a balanced, healthy body is *strengthening the muscles that are weak—in almost all cases it is the core muscles—and stretching the muscles that are tight, which are often the postural muscles of the hips, back and shoulders.* It's really that simple!

Core strength is important for all kinds of people and all forms of movement. While most of my students are active and healthy, some have come to me complaining of minor aches and pains. Together we were able to alleviate their pain by strengthening the core and stretching those muscles that had, in almost every case, never been stretched. It was a lot of hard work, but, in the end, we improved the quality of their lives, perhaps reducing the risk of more serious injury. These students are success stories. And then there are my relentless athletic types—marathon runners and competitive athletes that "got game" by focusing on strengthening their core, along with stretching their overworked muscles that often seized up from repetitive training. But don't worry. You don't have to bend like a yogi or have terminator type torsos to feel good. Just making some subtle shifts, as the majority of my students did, can help. Truthfully, many of them come to class once or twice a week just because it makes them feel good.

"I was a runner for over twenty years and never stretched. As a result, I experienced severe lower back pain and could not stand for more than ten minutes. After exhausting my medical options, my doctor suggested that I try core strength exercises. So I did and after five months my pain was reduced by almost ninety percent; it truly changed my life."

—KJEHL RASMUSSEN, ATTORNEY/MOVIE PRODUCER

"As a marathon runner and triathlete, I was continually plagued by back pain and leg injuries. I had done sit-ups in the gym off-and-on, but never really focused on 'core' training. When I began to work with Karon on shoulder, back, hip and abdominal stabilization, things really began to change. Now I am completing events without injury! Core training has changed my life. I am a better and happier athlete!"

—COREY SELF, COMPUTER SALES

When you consider skipping stretching or core strengthening exercises in order to shave a few minutes off your workout, think again! On one level, you are missing out on a valuable component of fitness that will ease muscle imbalances that can cause a wide variety of injuries, from shoulder strain to lower back pain. On another level, you'll miss out on a great opportunity to make your abs and midsection look trim and fit. Core weakness and muscle tightness will eventually take a toll on your good health and good looks. According to the latest thinking among sports medicine experts, you are missing out on the most critical part of fitness if you are not centering your workout around your core. But don't take my word for it:

"When people think of 'core' they think of abdominals, but core training includes musculature in the low back and pelvic floor as well. Core strength and endurance are essential to having good core stability and a healthy spine.

The healthier these areas are, the more likely it is that individuals will be able to carry on the activities of daily living and will be less susceptible to having low back pain. The reason we see a lot of adults with poor posture is because of weaknesses in these areas. If one's posture is exceptionally poor for periods of time, spinal structures can be weakened. This weakness is what leads to low back pain and some injuries."

—ERIN KLOEPFER, 50-PLUS MOMENTUM COORDINATOR'S ASSISTANT
AT THE BAYLOR TOM LAUNDRY FITNESS CENTER

"Core strength allows an athlete to maintain proper posture in the face of overwhelming fatigue. Correct posture reduces the energy cost of movement and permits more energy to be directed to the proper application of force."

—ROBERT VAUGHAN, PHD AT THE BAYLOR TOM LAUNDRY FITNESS CENTER

"Core strength is an absolute necessity for optimum performance from everyday activities to sports. Yet, the core is one of the least trained areas of our bodies. From early childhood to adulthood we continually ignore this essential aspect of fitness. And we pay the price through injury. As a physical therapist and fitness junkie, I have found core training to be the 'missing link' because it allows my patients and myself to return to maximum potential. It really works!"

—ROBIN BARRETT, PHYSICAL THERAPIST

"The core is where movement originates. If one had a weak core but big strong external/superficial muscles, it would be the same as having a drag car race engine placed in a Pinto car frame. The big race engine would not be able to reach its highest number of Rpm's or greatest power without the frame falling apart first."

—RYAN TOMPKINS, STRENGTH & CONDITIONING COORDINATOR
AT THE BAYLOR TOM LAUNDRY FITNESS CENTER

"I find that many individuals think their backs are weak. With a detailed evaluation, I often discover that the superficial back muscles along with the anterior shoulder muscles are actually overworked while the deep stabilizing muscles of the core are inactive. The key to active core conditioning is core education. Patients are often surprised at how much mental and physical effort is required to understand and learn core activation. Once they understand the key connections between the hips, pelvic floor and deep abdominals, all their exercises come to life. A deep understanding (pun intended) of core isolation can effect simple day to day activities as well as set the stage for enhanced sports performance."

—KAREN SANZO, PHYSICAL THERAPIST AND PILATES TEACHER TRAINER

As these experts attest, core strength will affect you in many ways at once. And as the new sports medicine science of prevention expands our understanding of how the body works at all levels, from the immune to neuromuscular systems, we will no doubt hear a lot more about the benefits of core strength. But there's still more ground to cover. So, let's go over some of the other benefits of core strength.

A BALANCED BODY

Depending on your lifestyle, workout habits and body alignment, certain muscle groups may work harder than others, creating imbalances in your body. Muscles work optimally when there is harmony between their length and tension relationship. In addition, if a muscle is too short or too long, then an imbalance can alter the relationship between the balanced system of muscle, tendon, fascia, and ligament. Tight muscles not only cause stiffness, aches, and pains, but may also stress the joints attached to the muscle pairing. When muscles move smoothly, so do the joints. Clearly, there is a synergistic action between these groups to keep you standing upright and moving well. When joint-muscle integrity is compromised, one group must overcompensate for the other. Whether through lifestyle choice, work habits, improper muscle training, or lack of body awareness (which I will address in detail in the next chapter), muscle imbalance happens. We all get caught up in the daily grind, never realizing that we're reshaping our bones and muscles and, thus, our posture. Most people work the typical eight-to-fourteen hour day, sitting around in positions that compromise their spine—slouching and hunching. A simple movement, such as always holding the telephone under your ear while talking, can alter your spine. If you wake up having no pain, but by the end of day are in pain, then it is time to make a few changes. Quitting work is not an option. But whether you lift, type, sit, or talk, you can keep your body healthy on the job and off by using what you learn here to alter your habits, beginning by training your muscles correctly.

CRUNCHES ARE OUT, CORE IS IN

Using your body the same way over and over again creates a muscle imbalance. You are, then, vulnerable to a number of things that can go wrong with your body: poor posture, aches and pains, or a major injury. Because your body works as a unit, muscle imbalance is often a result of how you move your body on a daily basis. Let's take the movement of an exercise we all know too well—the crunch. Most people have no idea that if you only do a crunch to strengthen your abs, then your core can actually weaken. If your core weakens, then your body can't hold itself upright correctly. When you can't sit or stand with good posture, then other muscle imbalances can happen, which can initiate the downward spiral of all kinds of aches and pains. Crunches are overrated and outdated! You wouldn't do a bicep curl to strengthen all the muscles in your arm, would you? Of course not! Why, then, strengthen all of your abdominal muscles with a crunch? When you over-strengthen the outer, or superficial, muscles of your abdomen, the deeper trunk stabilizing muscles weaken. This is the quintessential example of training the abdominals independently rather than strengthening the core as a whole. What this means to you is obvious—a belly pooch (now you know why you still have one) and perhaps some lower back tenderness. What makes matters worse is that you may not have fully strengthened the superficial muscles correctly at all.

It is important to pay attention to body alignment. For example, most people have overdeveloped and tight hip flexors, because they are the most frequently used muscles in the body. When tight, the psoas, which is a major hip flexor muscle, can pull on the lumbar vertebrae, upsetting the placement of the pelvis and causing the belly to bulge. If you train your abdominals in this bulging position, then you are repeatedly training your muscles in a shortened length. Or put another way: Building muscle on top of a bulging belly enhances just that—a bulging belly.

BENDING LIKE A YOGI

If you ignore your body as a whole, and consistently work out without regard for the end result for your entire body, then muscle imbalance and joint tension are very real possibilities. Similarly, muscle imbalances trigger a muscle tug-of-war between the tight, strong, superficial muscles and the sagging, weak deep stabilization muscles. To help adjust this imbalance, you must also stretch! Muscles fall into two categories, depending on how they function from day to day. Some muscles, for example, stabilize your body, while others move your body. Because many of us crave cardio and thrive on a "going-for-the burn" type of workouts while neglecting to stretch, we tend to train the most noticeable muscles, even as the smaller, lesser known stabilizing muscles go unnoticed and untrained. No doubt you know the big movement muscles: hamstrings, quadriceps, and the six-pack abdominals, just to name a few. But, in order to ease muscle imbalances, you should get to know the muscles that lie beneath those large muscle groups. *In this book, you will actively and consciously stretch all the muscles that affect core stability, many of which are ignored in most workouts. It's not enough to bend here and there, your goal is to stretch no fewer than two to three days a week.*

Obviously, strengthening your core is crucial to good health, for all the reasons I have already mentioned. But there's more! A strong core also helps you stretch correctly. *If your core is weak, then you will stretch the body incorrectly—out of alignment. When the body is not aligned, then you are only reinforcing muscle imbalances, reinforcing the downward cycle.* This happens all the time. In the gym, I continually see students stretching haphazardly. Let's take the quadriceps—the muscles that run up and down the front of your thigh. While stretching the quadriceps, the pelvis must remain stable while lifting the heel to the buttock. In many cases, though, students throw their bodies forward to grab the ankle, just to hold the stretch. This situation throws the pelvis out of alignment and minimizes a much-needed stretch. *Your pelvis must always remain stable in a stretch.* And a strong core helps hold your pelvis steady. Stretching, of course, has so many benefits, the least of which is that it just feels so good. Just as tight muscles leave you feeling tight, tense, and tortured, loose muscles leave you tranquil, comfortable, and relaxed.

Bending here and there is not enough—you must actively and consciously stretch! The body must be aligned for a stretch to be beneficial to your body, and it is important to hold each stretch for at least thirty seconds. If you don't lengthen the muscles, tendons, ligaments, and connective tissue to their full length at least three times a week, then they will gradually shorten. So stretch, bend, and twist!

Look Great at Any Age

Aging happens, and it begins as early as your twenties. But you don't have to rush it along. You can defy your age by exercising and eating right. *Even if you are only in your twenties, now is the time to launch an anti-aging strategy, such as a core strength program, because you are establishing healthy habits for life. Essentially, good health begins in your twenties and thirties.* So, the following is a decade-by-decade guide that tells you what changes happen at which point in life and the lifestyle changes to make now. Let's start with the fun-loving twenties. Aging starts with a few gray hairs, perhaps a thin spot. Your flexibility is somewhat compromised, if you had any in the first place. Emotionally and physically, you need to exercise to deal with the stress of getting your career off the ground. Now is a good time to start a core strength program because you are developing exercise habits that will last you the rest of your life. Pay attention to how you workout and your body form, because later in life you will begin to feel the results of bad workout habits, and poor posture. In your thirties, you may notice more gray hairs. Then the mysterious dimples start to appear on your thighs, attracting your full attention. The thirty-something man is usually able to pinch an inch, sometimes for the first time in his life. He is probably working long sedentary hours and not paying any attention to the love handles growing under his well tailored business suit. The thirty-something woman may be thinking about starting a family, and a balanced exercise routine, including core strength, makes pregnancy much more comfortable and healthier. And it makes getting her figure back after pregnancy much easier. In this decade, muscle atrophy begins to accelerate right under your clothes. You probably notice more aches and pains. Perhaps your lower back is acting up, which can be a direct result of sitting long hours a day.

The fabulous forties are not so fab! You must really work at keeping your body in shape. If you have been in denial, you are about to snap out of it because the most dramatic effects of aging start in this decade. Your muscles rebel; you can't lift as much, nor eat as much. And if you try, your body lashes out by growing stiffer and fatter. Your body deteriorates the most in your forties—it's here you will have to pay the most attention to your exercise and eating.

By age fifty, your bones are under attack; they are losing more and more calcium, thus becoming more brittle by the day. *In fact, bone density begins decreasing at a rate of 1% per year after 35 years old.* This pattern continues well into your seventies. By the time you hit seventy, you can lose a couple of inches in height as the vertebrae thin and shrink, adding girth to your middle.

It is not uncommon, then, that life changes bring people to exercise. *Whether you are in your twenties or eighties, core strength is the anti-aging answer.* There are dozens of studies that show that moving earlier in life and keeping your muscles strong can protect you from decades of decay. In addition, as you age, balance becomes a topic of great concern. After all, nobody wants to fall and injure themselves. This fear is backed by an alarming statistic. There are over 300,000 cases of broken hips treated in U.S. hospitals each year. Stability comes before mobility, which is why strengthening your core makes so much sense, especially as you age. By strengthening your core, you will significantly decrease the risk of falling and breaking or fracturing a bone, which could lay you up for several months.

STAYING STRONGER LONGER

How you age—whether you stay youthful, trim, and energetic—is largely up to you. Age alone does not tell the entire truth about someone; it does not determine how well you move or hold yourself, nor does it dictate how strong or how healthy you are. Age does not have to contribute to injury either; if they don't take care of themselves, individuals in their twenties can injure themselves just as easily as an older person. If you are looking for an exercise program to grow old with, then you have turned to the right book. There is no magic pill; exercise is a lifetime commitment to staying strong, healthy, and fit. Core strength can age you gracefully. Not only will you increase your energy, but you will also prevent some of the aches and pains associated with aging. For example, joint flexibility, the range of motion of a joint, decreases with age. Over time, you lose the ability to touch your toes or raise your arms over your head. Eventually you may not be able to scratch your back or turn your head to look behind you. But these limitations are not inevitable. With the exercises presented here you can maintain more of your strength and mobility throughout your life.

WISER WEIGHT LOSS

The Core Strength Workout will also control the extra inches that seem to appear out of nowhere. Your muscles get flabby not necessarily because of age, but more likely because you don't get off the couch. Probably the biggest benefit of this core strength program is that these exercises strengthen your body from head to toe. Fat does not burn as many calories as muscle does. You can slightly adjust your basal metabolic rate or BMR, the minimum amount of calories burned by your body, by increasing your muscle mass. So adding more muscle increases your calorie burn, which is the best way to trim inches and slim your body. Core strength exercises slow down age-related muscle loss as well. Here is a fact: An active person will decrease 0.5% physiologically per year; whereas, an inactive person or unfit person will decrease 2% per year. *One major misconception is that aging slows down your body's rate of calorie consumption; but it is lack of activity which depletes your muscle and decreases your BMR, not aging alone.*

WHAT'S SEX GOT TO DO WITH IT?

Core strength enhances your sex life—period! You can look forward to deeper orgasms, because doing exercises that contract your pelvic floor muscles, the multi-layered hammock-like muscles that run from your pubic bone to the coccyx, strengthens the muscles that are responsible for orgasms. Many women are told to do Kegel exercises, which is a contracting and releasing of the pelvic floors, during and post pregnancy to restore the strength in the pelvic floors. Some women suffer from an occasional incontinence, often following childbirth, which can be alleviated by these exercises as well. Men can benefit from Kegel for the same reasons. And with stronger pelvic muscles, your stamina will increase—reason for both you and your partner to celebrate!

MEN CAN BENEFIT FROM KEGEL TOO!

According to a team at the Kaiser Permanente Medical Center in Los Angeles, radical prostatectomy can cause temporary incontinence in up to 87% of the men who have the surgery. Dr. Sherif Aboseif, who led the study, instructed half the men to do Kegels twice a day after surgery while the other half got no specific instructions. "Overall 66 percent of the patients were continent at 16 weeks," Aboseif's team wrote. "But those who did their Kegels regained control earlier."

Reuters_News@reuters.com (June 27, 2003)

IF NOT NOW, WHEN?

Much of the value of this work is that it enhances the quality of your life. You can apply what you learn from these exercises to your total health regimen. It is not too early or too late to start thinking about ways to protect your health. Of course, this core strength program will not cure everything that ails you. Yet, you will benefit regardless of your age or fitness level. Staying stronger longer means that you will increase the odds of staying independent with the freedom to move and get about as you age. You will strengthen your body as a whole, increase flexibility, rebalance muscles groups that have often been neglected, and tighten your torso. With the core strength workout you can get curves that show off you shape, and strength that prepares you for anything life might throw your way!

Let's take one last look of the benefits of a hard core workout. A hard core:

Builds Strength

Eliminates muscle aches and pains, including those that result from joint stiffness

Improves Posture

Redistributes your weight

Stretches the body

Heightens energy levels—muscles will get stronger to support an active lifestyle

Improves balance

Trims your torso

Slows the aging process

Heightens sexual performance

Reduces fatigue

WRAPPING IT UP: CORE SECRETS

- Your core initiates movement. It extends from the base of your neck to the muscles between your legs and is made up of overlapping layers of muscles, consisting of all the muscles in your abdomen, back, hips, and pelvic floor.

- All movement begins with your core, which is why *The Core Strength Workout* is your first line of defense against pain and injury.

- If you are ignoring your core, then you are setting yourself up for all kinds of problems in life: flabby muscles, pot bellies, love handles, and muscle imbalances that can radiate soreness in the form of shoulder strain to lower back pain.

- To get a balanced, healthy body, use the exercises that follow, which will combine to strengthen your weak muscles and stretch your tight muscles.

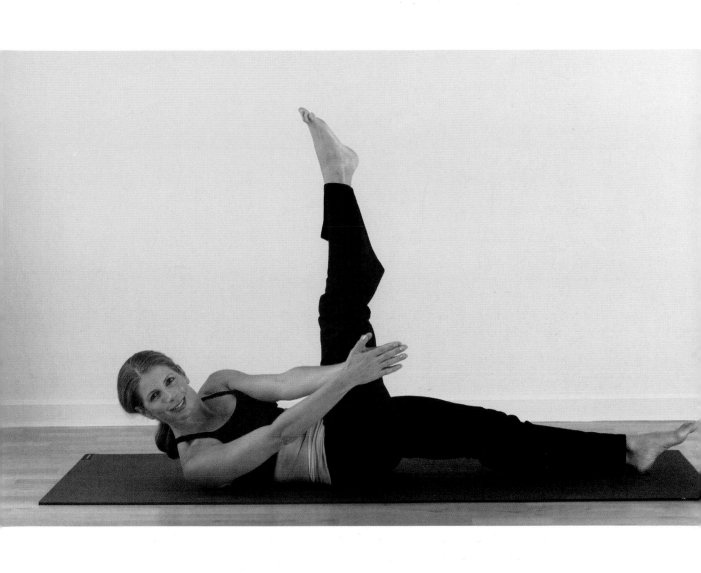

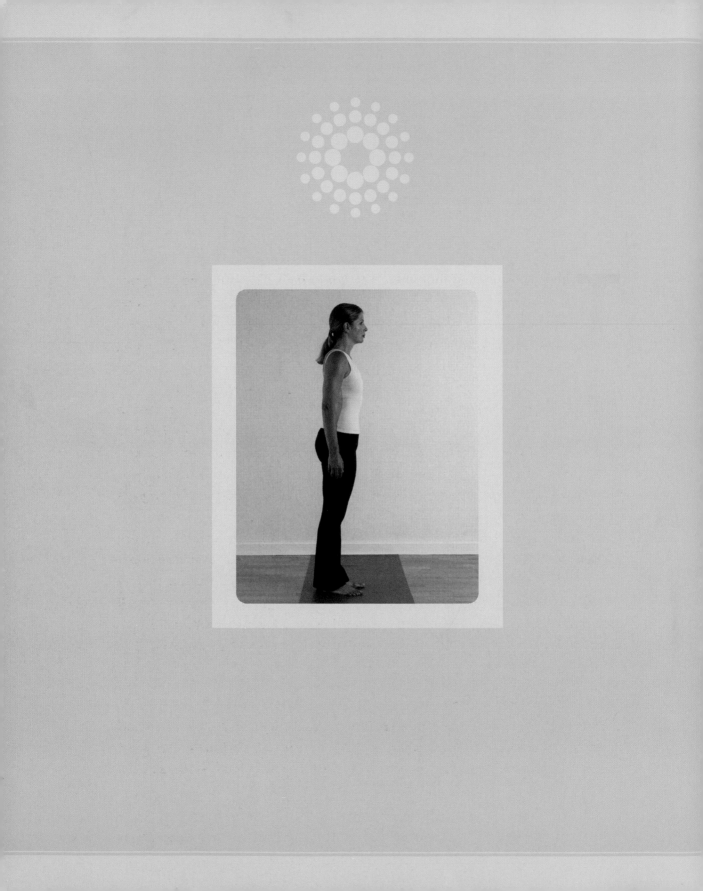

Chapter 2

Invisible Lift

There's posture and then there's *posture-luscious!* The latter radiates grace and poise and oozes sex appeal. It turns heads when entering a room. And while there's no such word, wouldn't we all love to have *posture-luscious?* Irresistibility isn't just about perfect abs or tight buns; it's about feeling really good in your own skin. It transcends the physical, sending the message that you are "queen of your world"! And all this begins with your posture.

Good posture projects health, vitality, and confidence. Plus, it can lessen the risk of all kinds of back woes. Poor posture alters your spine and its look, causing a lifetime of annoying aches and pains: muscle spasms in the lower back, decreased lung capacity, compressed nerves, chronic neck pain, and headaches. Of course, it won't soothe all of your aches and pains, but good posture is a necessary building block for health.

This chapter moves you toward your best body. For starters, you'll measure how you stand, right now. With that assessment, along with information about the muscles and bones that keep you upright, you can make the necessary postural corrections. Essentially, we're talking about body awareness! You'll hold your head a little higher, walk a bit taller, and exercise to become your utterly radiant self. If you like the sound of *posture-luscious,* then just wait.

BEATING THE BACK BLUES

Stand up straight and you exude confidence and good health; walk around slumping and you convey weakness and poor health. Individuals with good posture look healthier, thinner, and sexier, while individuals with less than perfect posture look dumpy and depressed. While bad posture equals bad backs, good posture beats the back blues. Stand tall and you will:

◇ look ten pounds lighter by trimming your waistline by an inch or so

◇ prevent back pain; poor posture is the leading cause of back pain

◇ grow an inch, or perhaps two

◇ have more energy, improving your day-to-day activities, which include lifting, walking, and exercising

---

THE SAD, SORE FACTS ABOUT BACKS!

Eighty percent of all adults will have back pain at some point in their lives; on any given day, an estimated 6.5 million people in the United States are bedridden due to back pain; and approximately 1.5 million new cases of back pain are seen by physicians each month. Back pain is the leading cause of visits to the doctor, of surgery, hospitalization, and work disability. Aching backs add up to $50 billion in medical costs annually in the United States.

If you slouch, you risk having all kinds of back pain. In fact, consider yourself lucky if back pain has not already become a constant in your life. Most adults are not so lucky. Muscles spasms, compressed nerves, and chronic headaches send more people to the doctor each year than the common cold. Lower back pain leaves more people throbbing than the common headache. Back injuries are also the leading cause of on-the-job injuries in adults. Not only are back problems painful, but they are also extremely expensive to recuperate from.

You don't have to take this lying down, though. Yes, your back may be defenseless against everyday physical demands; activities such as sitting, bending, and twisting cause wear and tear on your back. If your back muscles are weak, it exasperates the wear and tear on your back and its supporting structure—the muscles, bones and ligaments. Strengthening your core, which includes both the abdominal and back muscles, helps you stay injury free.

STACKING YOUR BACK

Since pain and poor posture go hand and hand, it's important to understand the amazing network of ligaments, muscles, and bones that keep you standing tall. For starters, your spine, also called the vertebral column, keeps you upright. Its bony blocks, or vertebrae, stack up on top of one another, twenty-six bones tall. Each vertebra is attached to its neighbor by three joints. While the vertebra provide back stability, the joints guide movement and provide flexibility. Your vertebrae are held together by a complex system of ligament, cartilage, and muscle. Ligaments are fibrous bands that hold the joints together, connecting bone to bone. Cartilage is the smooth tissue on the ends of the bones that allows the joints to move easily. The muscles that protect the spine are designed to pull equally; they contract or lengthen in a coordinated manner to keep you standing and moving smoothly.

The body's shock absorbers, called discs, are plump pieces of cartilage that act as cushions for the vertebra as you run, walk and move. Only when the spine is lined up correctly, with musculoskeletal integrity, can this network work with precision. However, pain, or an injury can strike any one of these elements, at any time: ligaments and tendons strain or rip, muscles tear or pull, joints wear out, and discs can rupture simply by lifting a heavy object. Standing correctly and strengthening and stretching your core muscles help to prevent such injuries.

Healthy backs have three natural curves. The first is at the neck, the cervical curve, and is made up of the first seven vertebrae (C1-C7), beginning at the base of your neck and continuing to the upper back. From there, the thoracic curve, consisting of twelve vertebrae, T1-T12, shapes the middle of your spine. And finally, the lumbar curve, or lower back, contains only five vertebrae, L1-L5, but it is the most susceptible to pain because it bears most of your body weight. Following these three curves come the sacral vertebrae, S1-S5, which act as one unit to create a flat bone, the sacrum, that rests on the base of your buttocks. And, finally, the coccygeal vertebrae, which are four immovable bones fused together to form your tailbone.

Muscles compensate to meet the demands of your life. As a general rule, when one set of muscles pulls too hard or not hard enough, then its pairing muscles must work that much harder to compensate. If your bones don't stack up correctly, then neither do your muscles, which leads to muscles that are too tight or too weak. This muscle imbalance puts extra wear and tear on your joints and the rest of your body. Friction, inflammation, and chronic pain can leave you feeling back-pain blue, and with a lighter wallet after all the doctor's and chiropractor's bills. But core strength exercises and better posture through body awareness can prevent most of these problems. The first step is to identify possible warning signs of trouble. Then stop or alter whatever activity is causing you pain and irritation. After that, you can begin to slowly and carefully find activities to improve your movement. Yes, you will stretch what needs to be stretched and strengthen what is weak in the coming chapters. But even more important, you need to develop body awareness to keep track of your posture and alignment throughout life.

THE MILITARY POSTURE

Much of the lumbar spine is vulnerable to injury because the area between your pelvis and low back holds most of your body weight. If your back is weak, that only makes things worse. Since the pelvis and lumbar spine directly influence what happens in the rest of the spine, take a good look at your lumbar curve.

A healthy lumbar spine has a slight arch, but a severe exaggeration of the lumbar curve, or lordosis, can cause major back problems. If your low back hikes your behind in the air and puffs out your chest, you have just enlisted yourself for some serious back woes. A combination of tight lower back muscles and weak abdominals is one of the primary causes of this over-exaggerated lumbar curve. This muscle struggle pulls your pelvis into a forward position, or anterior tilt, because the tight (not necessarily strong) back muscles usually overpower the weak abdominals. If you are unsure whether you fall into this category, try standing against a wall. Place the back of your shoulders and buttocks on the wall. The palm of your hand should fit between you and the wall. If you can slide your fist back and forth, then you may have too much arch. Pay attention to these warning signs:

- You may experience dull, aching or shooting pains in your lower back.

- You may lock your knees while standing, which puts added pressure on your legs as well as your back.

- Too much lumbar curve may also force you to turn your feet in, causing you to balance the bulk of your body weight on your big toe rather than over your entire foot.

- You may also have tense, tight, lifted shoulders and a puffed out chest that will weaken your upper back muscles.

- You may have muscle imbalance. The abdominals lengthen and become weak while the back muscles shorten in length—becoming tense and tight and throwing off the alignment of the pelvis.

- You may develop compression of the sciatic nerve, resulting in pain or numbness that radiates down your leg.

THE FLAT BACK POSTURE

Similar lower back problems happen when the lumbar arch is completely eliminated. This time, the pelvis tilts back, locking into a pelvic tilt position so the back looks completely flat. Believe it or not, the flat back posture is common among athletes—mainly because they don't stretch. Runners, tennis players, and tri-athletes all tend to have tight hamstrings, which eventually pulls the back of the pelvis down, wiping out the natural arch. However, athletic types are not the only ones that need to worry. If you are chained to a keyboard or desk, sitting for long periods of time without getting up, or if you rarely stretch, then you are equally helpless against tightness, and pain. Test yourself by standing against a wall. Place your shoulders and buttocks against the wall. If you can't slide your hand between your lower back and the wall, then you might have a flat back. Warning signs are:

- You may experience chronic lower back tightness due to tight hamstrings and hips.

- You may hang your head forward, overstretching the muscles of the cervical spine.

- You may, in addition to hanging your head forward, round your shoulders. This begins the downward cycle of altering the curve of the upper spine.

- You may have a muscle imbalance that consists of tight hamstrings and hips, while the abdominals are short and tight.

THE SLUMP POSTURE

Perhaps in your teens you rounded your shoulders, trying in vain not to tower over your friends in high school. Maybe your work keeps you slumping over piles of papers. Whatever the cause, you are compromising the alignment of your upper spine, and often your neck. Slumping slowly changes the curve of your thoracic spine. An exaggerated curve in the thoracic spine is called kyphosis. A series bone disease called osteoporosis can also round the upper spine. In fact, this curve could be your only sign that you are losing bone density, because osteoporosis is often called the silent disease—it has no symptoms.

A common pattern with this problem are short and tight chest muscles with long and weak upper back muscles. If so, the upper back muscles can become so frail that they do not have the strength to hold you in an upright position. Even worse, the muscles in the front of your body, including your abdominals, will also have the tendency to shorten in length, causing your rib cage to compress toward your hips. This reduces your breathing capacity. If your upper back feels tight and tense most days, then take a look at your upper back curve. Warning signs are:

- You may physically drop an inch or two in height just by rounding your shoulders.

- You may, at the same time, add an inch or two width-wise to your mid-section as the rib cage compresses toward your hips.

- You may not have the chest size you once enjoyed—men or women!

- You may not breathe as deeply because of rib cage compression.

- You may have tight, tense shoulders and upper back pain.

- You may experience cervical compression, chronic neck tension, and headaches.

- You may have a muscle imbalance of weak, lengthened upper back muscles and short, tight chest muscles.

IS YOUR HEAD ON STRAIGHT?

As you look at your spine, take notice of the position of your head. If your shoulders round forward, then your head probably hangs forward as well. Your head is designed to sit directly on top of your spine; this is a neutral position that reduces neck and back pain and improves your posture. How you hold and move your head can directly alter the supporting structure in your spine, because your head weighs about ten to fourteen pounds. Even if your head is only slightly off-balance, you may eventually alter the curve of the upper back, which can cause spasms as the extra weight makes the neck muscles work that much harder. A good point to remember is that the spine begins between your ears. Ideally, then, your head should line up directly over your shoulders. Good alignment begins here, with a balanced relationship among your head, neck and shoulders. If your head is not straight, then the length of your spine may shrink due to the downward spinal compression: a forward hanging head rounds the shoulders and then the shoulders compress the rib cage, which results in lost inches in your spine and your height. Warning signs are:

- You may experience strain and pain in the back of the neck, as the added weight puts pressure on the joints and nerves.

- You may have chronic pain from cervical compression with symptoms varying from a stiff neck to tingling or numbness in the arms and hands.

- You may suffer from chronic tension headaches.

Battling Brittle Bones

Osteoporosis is not only found among the elderly. You might not think that you are at risk, but early signs of osteoporosis, or low bone density, can be found in women in their twenties and thirties. *Regardless of your age, you need to consider an anti-brittle bone campaign, before osteoporosis alters your posture and appearance, and possibly even changes how you can live your life.*

As you age, bone production slows down; your bones lose the ability to rebuild themselves. Bone regeneration starts to slow in your thirties and decelerates as you approach menopause, when the ovaries stop producing estrogen. In fact, women can lose up to 20% of their bone mass in the first five to seven years following menopause. Nearly 40% of postmenopausal women have osteopenia, the early signs of osteoporosis. As the bones lessen in density and become thin and brittle, you become more susceptible to fractures. This decay or bone loss is a direct result of the natural aging process and the lifestyle choices we make. In other words, we can slow it down.

Bones are alive and continually regrowing, so you possess the power to nurture them with what you eat and how you exercise. Your bones are made of collagen and calcium. Collagen is a glue-like matter made up of vitamin C and water that is a part of most structures of the body: skin, bones, teeth, blood vessels, cartilage, tendons and ligaments. Calcium is a mineral that is stored in the bones so it can be used whenever it is needed for many of the vital body functions. As the bones give up calcium, the body replaces the loss. The body always needs calcium and will recruit it from other bones when the supply is low. A deficit, then, affects how bones are remade. Osteoporosis is often called the silent disease because there are no symptoms, but it usually shows up first as back pain. *Signs of osteoporosis can be as little as rounded shoulders or back pain between the lower borders of the shoulder blades, or as severe as a hump in the upper back. This hump, called Dowager's hump, affects 40% of the women who have osteoporosis. It is important to be clear: Osteoporosis is an insidious disease that alters your posture; it is not caused by poor posture.*

OSTEOPOROSIS FACTS AND FIGURES

Osteoporosis is a major public health threat for an estimated 44 million Americans. In the U.S. today, 10 million individuals are estimated to already have the disease and almost 34 million more are estimated to have low bone mass leading to osteoporosis. Of the 10 million, 8 million are women and 2 million are men. One in two women and one in four men over age 50 will have an osteoporosis-related fracture in their lifetime, including hip, vertebra, and wrist fractures. Osteoporosis is responsible for more than 1.5 million fractures annually. The estimated national direct expenditures (hospitals and nursing homes) for osteoporotic and associated fractures was $17 billion in 2001 ($47 million each day, and the cost is rising).

Facts and Figures are from the National Osteoporosis Foundation

---

By now, you probably know that low calcium intake depletes your bones. But there are other factors—ones you may not know of—that put you at risk for osteoporosis. Answer the questions below. Depending on how many "Yes" responses you have to the questions below, you may be on your way to having bone problems. Now is a good time to evaluate your risk and then take control. Are you at risk?

- Do you weigh less than 127 pounds?

- Are you postmenopausal or have you undergone surgery to induce menopause?

- Are you fair skinned, Caucasian, Asian, or of Scandinavian origin?

- Do you have a small body frame with low body weight, or are you underweight? Do you have a history of anorexia?

- Have you or a member of your immediate family ever broken or fractured a bone as an adult?

- Are you sedentary?

- Do you smoke?

- Is your diet low in dairy products, or very high in processed food like vending machine snacks, canned goods, or white bread?

- Do you regularly drink alcohol, coffee and/or cola drinks?

- Does osteoporosis run in you family, or does your mother have osteoporosis?

The more questions you answered "Yes" to, the higher your relative risk of osteoporosis. If you feel that you may be at risk for osteoporosis, contact the National Osteoporosis Foundation (202-223-2226) for more information. In the meantime, there are things you can do to protect yourself from this disease.

Your risk for developing osteoporosis can be greatly reduced by making specific lifestyle choices. For one thing, if you smoke, stop! After kicking the smoking habit, in your twenties, thirties, and forties you can act proactively to prevent osteoporosis by building your bones through a diet high in calcium and plenty of exercise. The good news is that experts have agreed on what type of exercise is best for your bones. Weight-bearing activity is most beneficial, meaning exercise that works against the force of gravity, like walking, running, climbing stairs and resistance training. Weight-bearing exercises, which include the core exercises in this book, are good for you because they involve movement that pulls on the bones as they work against gravity, thus triggering more bone production and increasing skeletal mass. Plus, weight bearing exercises may enhance mineral absorption. Exercise also slows the rate of bone loss, which can help prevent fractures and disfiguring changes in your posture. A strong core will also help prevent fractures by enhancing balance, increasing strength, and developing coordination.

My Aching Joints: Arthritis

Perhaps you know the feeling—that stiffness when you get out of bed in the morning. Your joints are not quite awake yet; they protest every slow step you take. What if you had to battle that stiffness around the clock? Sadly, many people do. *Arthritis or joint inflammation is a disease that can strike in your twenties, thirties, or forties.* And, yet again, the alignment of your bones along with the working muscles is your first defense against the debilitating disease.

Approximately 70 million Americans have arthritis, according to the Arthritis Foundation. Arthritis, or cartilage degeneration, causes inflammation or swelling in the joints because as the cartilage deteriorates, the bones rub together, which can be extremely painful depending on the type of arthritis.

But while some forms of arthritis are hereditary, prevention is still key for most kinds of arthritis. How you exercise, how you work, and how you eat all play a major role in the development of arthritis. Proper alignment, movement, and nutrition are key to maintaining your overall health and preventing arthritis. You know that misalignment and muscle imbalance can cause wear and tear on your joints. For example, let's say that you round your shoulders. Over time, your pectoral muscles in your chest shorten and become more dominant while your upper back muscles lengthen or outstretch. This muscle pairing pulls unequally because the over-stretched back muscles become weaker than the pairing chest muscles. Eventually, the attached joint, which is the axis of movement, may rub, causing a popping sound as a result of the stress on the joint. You must align, align and align, whether you are sitting at a desk, walking down the street or pumping weights in the gym.

You must also move, move and move! Of course, if you are aching and in pain, exercising is the last thing you want to do. Yet research shows that activity keeps the pain at bay, de-stiffens the joints, improves the functions of the joints and, most importantly, strengthens the joints' supportive structures. With a little help from you, joints can maintain their full function throughout your life. For example, as you age, the ligaments and tendons lose elasticity and the joints cannot function in a full range of motion. *Full range of motion (ROM) is the degree to which a limb can move around a joint without wear and tear on surrounding parts of the body, including the joints.* Over time, they become inflexible. Stretching can do a lot to maintain joint flexibility.

Exercising without stressing your joints is equally important. For example, training the body as a whole, rather than one muscle at a time, helps create symmetry within your body. It is important to strengthen your muscles equally so the surrounding joints are protected, which is why body awareness—how you hold your body while exercising or just running errands during the day—is vital to joint health.

SELF-EVALUATION: STACKING UP YOUR BONES

As I've explained above, posture matters! Bad posture, though, may feel right to you. So, you must make subtle changes every day to re-learn what good posture feels like. Stacking your bones correctly is the easiest and cheapest way to ward off pain. Before wrapping up this chapter, I will show you how to evaluate your own posture. First you will take before-training pictures and then pictures after eight weeks of training. That way, you can have a point of reference—"before" and "after" pictures that measure your progress. You may want to ask a loved-one to take these pictures of you because you need to take them with your clothes off. The idea is to reveal as much of your body as possible. Be truthful so you can make improvements from here. You don't have to pose, just take a deep breath and stand as casual as possible! Take a front, side and back view, several shots of each. Review the pictures and have a piece of paper and pencil ready to write down your thoughts. Ask yourself these questions:

- Does your head hang forward?

- Are you slumping over—shoulders and upper back rounded forward?

- Are your shoulders nearing your ears?

- Is one shoulder higher than the other?

- Does your abdomen bulge?

- Does your lower back have a severe arch?

- Do you lock your knees while standing?

- Do your ankles roll in, causing the arches in your feet to flatten; or roll out, causing you to put pressure on the outside portion of your feet?

Now, compare your posture to what is considered good posture:

- Your ears, shoulders and hips are in line.

- Your head sits directly on top of your shoulders.

- Your shoulders are not slumped.

- Your shoulder blades lie flat against your back, not winging out or sticking up from your spine.

- ⟨⟩ Your chest is open, not sunken or compressing the rib cage down toward the hips. Your rib cage should look broader at the top and taper as it draws closer to the hips.

- ⟨⟩ Your arms hang directly at your side with your palms facing toward your body.

- ⟨⟩ Your pelvis sits evenly on the hip bones, no tilting.

- ⟨⟩ Your bottom is not tucked underneath you or sticking out in the air; the lumbar spine has a slight natural curve.

- ⟨⟩ Your upper thighs are slightly rotated out.

- ⟨⟩ Your knees are soft, not locked into position. Each kneecap is approximately in line with the middle toe of the foot.

- ⟨⟩ Your feet stand evenly on the floor, no rolling in or out.

- ⟨⟩ Your back should have three noticeable curves to evenly distribute your body weight.

- ⟨⟩ Your face should be relaxed, especially the jaw. And smile!

POSTURE TRANSFORMATION

The goal of achieving proper alignment is to heed the signs early, before a full-blown problem develops. Posture does matter, and fixing it now is probably the cheapest and least invasive form of preventative medicine. The best way to improve your posture is to properly align your body. Every time you consciously align your body, you are reinforcing good posture and training your body as to what good posture feels like. These core exercises to come, then, can play a vital roll in enhancing your posture and your life—you just have to get started.

WRAPPING IT UP: CORE SECRETS

- ☼ Good posture can make you look ten pounds lighter by instantly trimming your waistline by an inch or so and adding an inch or two to your height.

- ☼ Bad posture is the leading cause of back pain. Stacking your bones correctly is the easiest and cheapest way to ward off back pain.

- ☼ Muscle spasms, compressed nerves, and chronic headaches send more people to the doctor each year than the common cold.

- ☼ Poor posture is more than just not standing up straight. When the bones are not aligned correctly, neither are the muscles. The effect is muscle imbalance, which can lead to friction, inflammation, chronic pain, and costly medical problems.

- ☼ Regardless of your age, you need to consider an anti-brittle bone campaign. *Early signs of osteoporosis can be found in women in their twenties and thirties.*

- ☼ 10 million individuals are estimated to already have osteoporosis. Of the 10 million, 8 million are women and 2 million are men.

- ☼ Experts agree on what type of exercise is best for your bones—weight bearing activity, exercises that work against the force of gravity, like walking, running, climbing stairs, and resistance training.

- ☼ Arthritis or joint inflammation is not just a disease of the elderly. Rather, it is a disease that can strike in your twenties, thirties, or forties. Core strength, proper alignment, and flexible muscles and joints may help prevent arthritis.

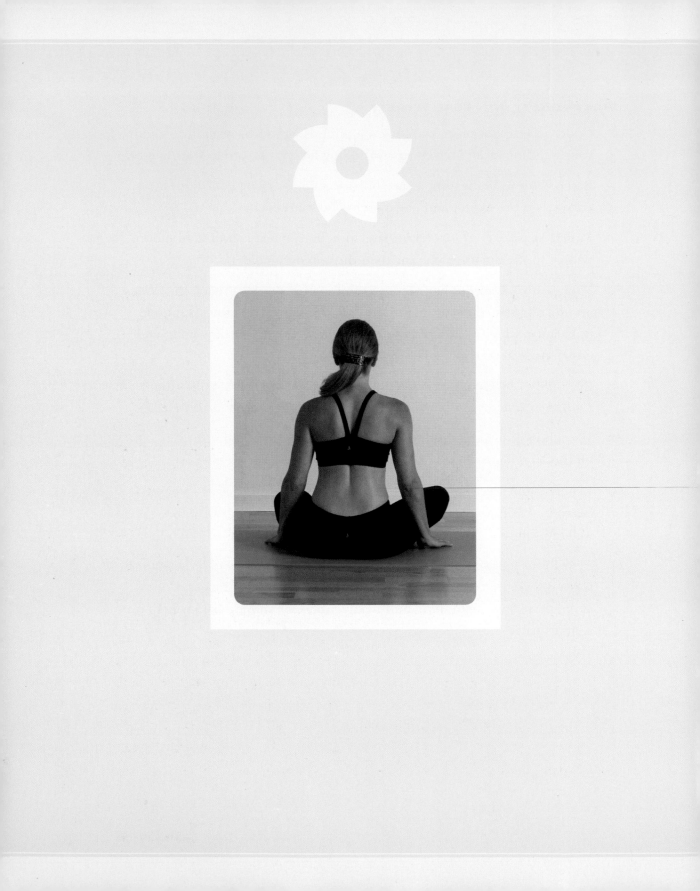

Chapter 3

Core Concepts

You feel pretty good, but sense that you could feel even better. Maybe you're dreaming of squeezing into your skinny jeans. Perhaps you're inches away from touching your toes for the first time since grade school. Possibly those body twinges keep you stiff and cranky—stealing precious moments from your life. As you inch toward your fitness goals, the questions remain: How will I age with grace and good health? How can I live my life to its fullest? Am I willing to do what it takes to enrich my life? If you've gotten this far, the answer is probably "Yes." Since you've accepted that core strength is lacking in your life, you are willing to set aside a little time, every day, to build the body you want. Yet, trying something new is daunting—it's so much easier to do what you always do. Right?

The truth is, engaging your deep core takes patience and motivation. What works is a combination of re-educating your mind and retraining your body; it's slowing down in each movement and thinking about what you're doing, rather than just going through the motions. This chapter, then, offers crucial core concepts so you can do the core exercises of this book safely. In addition, I include some mini-exercises that can help you find limitations in your own body—perhaps the ones you've found while evaluating your posture—and how to correct them. By watching and feeling what's happening in your body, without judgment, you can take yourself to a place of observation where you accept the things you can't change about your body and change what you can! By admitting your body's flaws (and we all have them), this work becomes about what you can do to lessen them, rather than simply an exercise routine.

My goal is to ease your learning process by showing you how to work sanely within your body and its limits. As you inch toward your goals, think about what really matters to you—whether it be enhancing your athletic performance, becoming pain free, or strutting your stuff wearing those skinny jeans.

A Core in Progress: Zip It Up

Core strength plays a daily role in your life: sitting at your desk, digging in the garden, carrying the groceries, opening a heavy door, lunging for a fallen glass, skiing a vertical slope, catching yourself in mid-fall—the list goes on and on. Strengthening your core, which includes both the abdominal and back muscles, provides support and protection for your spine. So imagine the core region as you get to know the overlapping and zigzagging muscles that contour your core.

Core strength begins with the deepest abdominal muscle, the transversus abdominis or transverse; its depth and location serve as an anatomical "wrap" around the trunk, forming a girdle of support and protection for your spine. This is why activating your transverse is the heart of this work. To feel your transverse contract, kneel on the floor or sit or stand in a comfortable position. Place your hands on your rib cage. Now force a cough. Did your feel your belly pull toward your spine? Did your rib cage move, shrinking your mid-section? If so, that's your transverse drawing in, as if a belt is tightening around your waist. In every exercise, imagine that belt buckling tighter and tighter to activate your transverse. *When you use your transverse correctly, your abdomen "hollows," as if forming the letter "C."* If not, then your belly may pop out like a loaf of bread. Never, ever give into this bulge. Always center your workout by focusing on an inward pull from the pubic bone to your navel. With this mini-exercise, you should feel the transverse engage.

Heel Slide

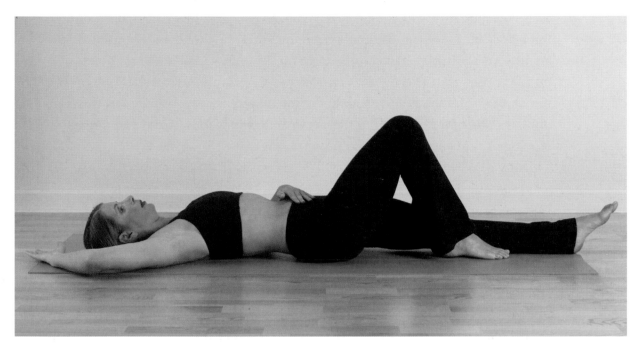

1 Lie down on your back, legs extended. Place the palm of your hand on your abdomen. Take a breath, and as you exhale, slide your heel into a bent knee position. As you exhale completely, you should begin to feel the inward pull and contraction of the transverse—remember to pull your navel in toward your spine the whole time. Your pelvis should not move an inch. Your lower lumbar spine must remain in neutral, with a slight arch. Perform ten slow repetitions with each leg.

Sitting on top of your transverse is the oblique system, which is divided into two sets of crisscrossing layers. These muscles criss-cross your abdomen to stabilize your core and give you your curves. They also let you flex, twist, and bend at the waist. To outline the direction of the external obliques, lay your hands along your waist, fingers down, as if you're putting your hands in your pant's pockets. Turn your fingers the opposite way to outline the internal obliques— remember, these muscles rest deep between your transverse and the external obliques. Imagine a letter "X" crisscrossing your body while bending and twisting at the waist to feel these muscles contract.

And finally, the most superficial muscle—the rectus abdominis. In combination with your external oblique muscles, it shapes the "six-pack" look. The rectus muscle runs up and down the length of your torso and flexes your spine. To feel this muscle contract, bend forward as if doing a crunch.

Just like the front, your back has its own set of overlapping muscles to protect and support your spine. The most common are the erector spinae, or gutter muscles, that run the length of your lumbar spine—from the sacrum to the last two thoracic vertebrae. Collectively, they arch your spine backward, which is known as a spine extension. There's also a deep, lesser known muscle, the multifidus, which runs almost the entire length of the spine from the sacrum to the cervical vertebrae. This muscle is mainly responsible for extension and rotation of your spine. Along with co-contractions from the transverse, this muscle is a major player in core stability.

The pelvic floors are the final set of core muscles. Contracting your pelvic floors, in conjunction with your abs and back muscles, creates hip and spinal stability. Your pelvic floor muscles not only provide pelvis support, but also prevent your organs from dropping to the floor, literally. The pelvic floors consist of five layers of fascia and muscles that cross through the bottom of the pelvis, from the pubic bone to the coccyx (anus). Imagine a hammock. It's a little hard to visualize, I know. But here's what I tell my students in class: Imagine squeezing into your favorite newly washed and dried jeans. Yes, these jeans are tight. So you pull your pubic bone to your navel and then your belly button in and up under your rib cage to zip them up—that zip begins between your legs with your pelvic floor muscles. If while in the restroom you were to try to stop the urine mid-stream, that would engage the same muscles.

So, as you can see, there are many muscles that make up your core. The idea is to start thinking about those muscles while doing these exercises, so you can work safely toward your goals.

FINDING NEUTRAL PELVIS

Healthy backs have three natural curves. To maintain those curves, you will work in what's called a neutral spine position, because it decreases the risk of injury by putting the least amount of stress on your body. It's vital to your shape—and health—to know how to move in and out of a neutral spine position. While many muscles and bones contribute to shaping your spine, there are two central parts: the hip-pelvis complex and the shoulder-scapula complex. Both must remain stable, or in a neutral position, before any movement can begin in your body. This comes down to a balancing act, literally, between body awareness and core training. Any limitation, muscle imbalance, inflexibility or weakness in your body can make holding a neutral spine difficult. But, don't worry. There are ways to get your bones moving in the right direction.

Let's begin with the hip and pelvis complex, which is the interconnected area of your hips, lower back, and pelvis. Its position is key to maintaining neutral spine because these muscles and bones directly interact with the spine and influence the position of your pelvis, which plays a major roll in lumbar stability. So, take your time looking at the position of your pelvis (you may need to review chapter two for posture tips). Here's a trick for finding a neutral pelvis in your own body: Think of your pelvis as a bowl filled to the brim with water. Over arching your lower back spills the water all over your feet, while a flat lower back drips the water down the back of your legs. In a neutral position, the bowl sits perfectly even, balancing the water inside the bowl. *In all exercises in this book, you'll always work with a neutral spine, keeping the pelvis in neutral.*

Practice Finding a Neutral Pelvis

by Rocking Your Pelvis

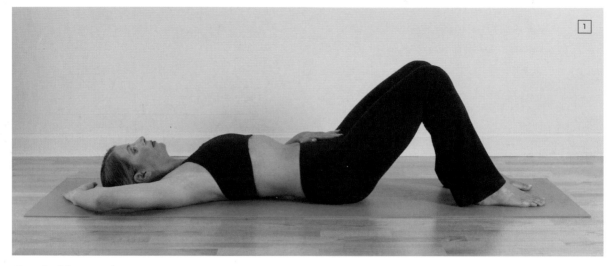

Neutral pelvis

1 To find a neutral pelvis, lie on your back and bend your knees. Place your hand, palm down, between your pubic bone and the bony protrusion of your pelvis. Point your fingers toward your pubic bone while resting the palm of your hand on the hip bone. When the pelvis is stable and neutral, your hand will lie flat; it's okay to have a natural arch in this position.

2 In a pelvic tilt, however, your lower back presses into the floor, so no light shines through your back and the floor. As the lumbar curve vanishes, the hand placement will shift—your fingertips will rest in a higher position than the palm of your hand.

3 Now, move the other way. Drop your tailbone to the floor, creating a huge lumbar arch. This anterior tilt will now move the palm of your hand higher than your fingers. Experiment. Rock your pelvis back and forth (which feels very good) and then try to return to a neutral position.

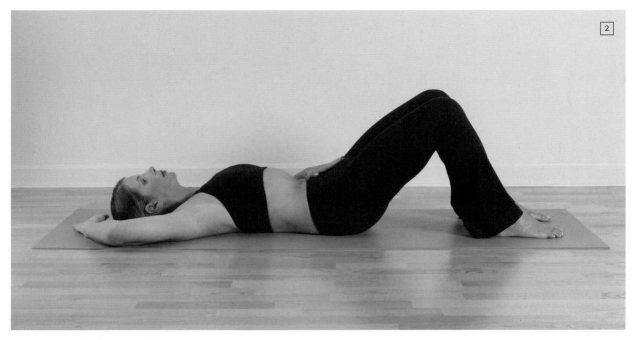

In a pelvic tilt, the fingertips lift higher than the palm of your hand.

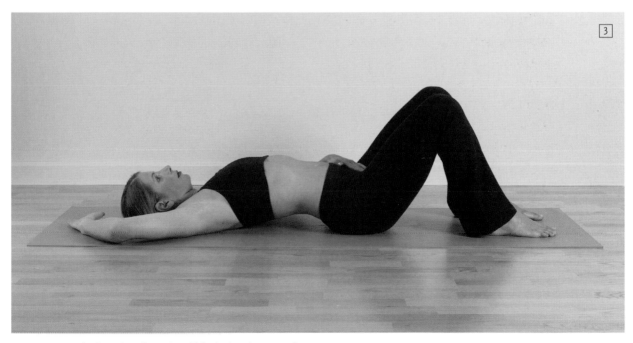

In an anterior tilt, the palm of your hand lifts higher than your fingertips.

Any muscle tightness around the pelvis can throw off its alignment. Here are two common muscle imbalances to look for: If you have tightness in the hamstrings and hips, then the pelvis may lock into a flat back position, eliminating the natural curve of your low back; tightness in the quadriceps and hip flexors, on the other hand, might shift the pelvis the other way, causing it to hyperextend the lumber curve. In either case, if your core muscles are weak, then controlling your pelvis is virtually impossible, which aggravates back matters.

Too much arch in the lower back is very obvious. Tight hamstrings and a flat back, however, are not so obvious. The test below can help you figure things out, plus it's a nice stretch. First, sit on the floor with your legs out straight. Sit directly on top of your sitz bones, or butt-bones, straightening your legs out in front of you. Don't lock your knees. Try to ground your butt-bones into the earth by grabbing the flesh from underneath your behind and pulling it away from the bones. Now pull the navel to the spine and sit up out of your hips. Don't forget to engage your pelvic floors by contracting between your inner thighs. This mini-exercise serves as both a test for tightness in your hamstrings and a hamstring stretch. If this is difficult, then you probably have some tightness in your hamstrings and you may have a hard time maintaining a neutral pelvis as well.

Hamstring Stretch

A Test for Tightness in the Hamstrings

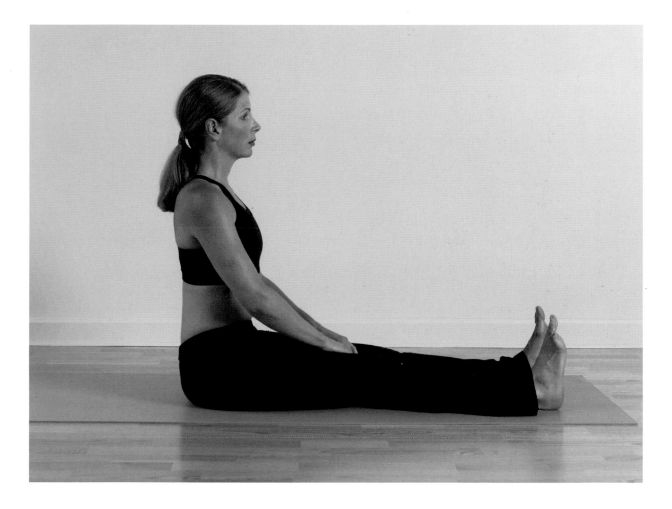

1 To find a centered position, pull the flesh away from your butt-bones, so you can sit directly on top of them.

(Hamstring Stretch, continued)

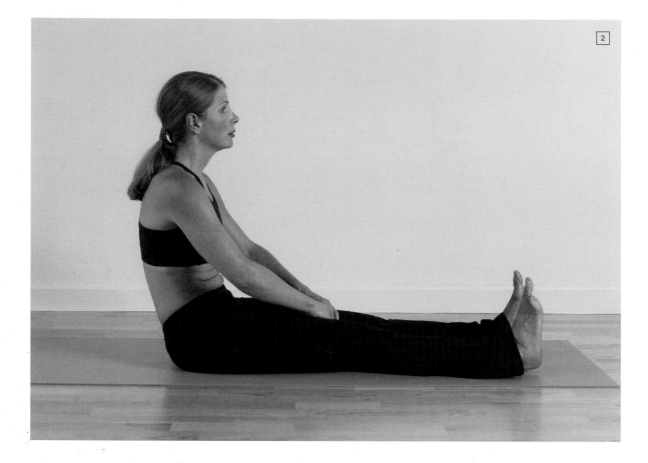

2 This is an example of tightness in the hips and hamstrings. As you can see, this position puts extra pressure on your lower spine.

3 If you can't maintain a slight arch in your lower lumbar in this position, then work with a small pad or rolled up blanket underneath your bottom to give your pelvis a little lift.

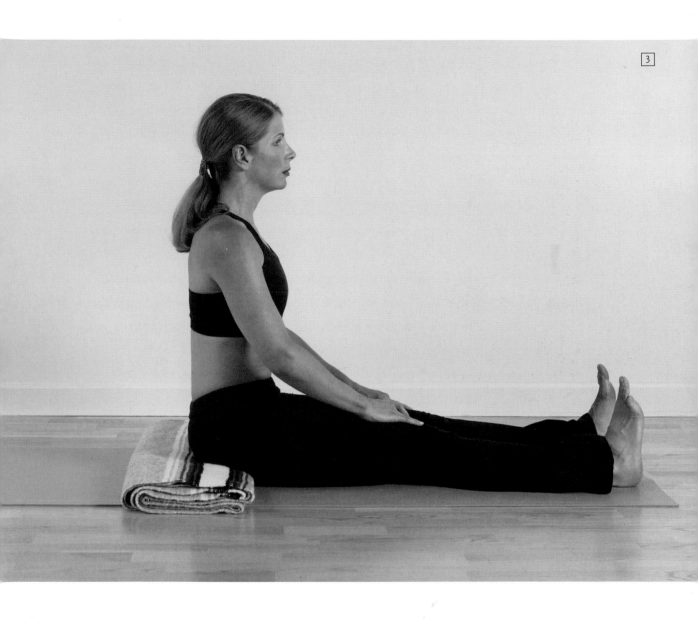

3

DECOMPRESSING YOUR HEAD, NECK AND SHOULDERS

It's not easy; upper back awareness takes practice. You may have tight chest muscles and weak upper back muscles, so strengthening will take time. Meanwhile, you can decompress your neck and enjoy a soothing moment by learning to relax your shoulders. For starters, hold a set of one- or two-pound dumbbell weights in each hand. Lift your shoulders to your ears and then lower them, letting the weights pull the shoulder blades down your back. Keep lifting your breastbone, so you don't round your shoulders and collapse into your chest. To gain awareness of your shoulder position, rotate your thumbs outward and inward to feel the rotation in the shoulder girdle. To create a neutral shoulder position, point your thumbs up toward the ceiling to gently contract the muscles underneath your arm-pits, then draw your shoulder blades slightly together and down your back. If your chest muscles are tight, you can use a stability ball to get a nice, deep stretch. Start by sitting on the ball, holding your weights in your hands, and then gradually slide your bottom off until your lower back is supported by the ball. Open your arms to the side. You should feel the stretch across your chest and arms as well.

Shoulder Savvy: Liberate Your Ears

Give yourself a hug! Do you feel the winged bones that protrude from your back? These bones are your shoulder blades, technically called the scapula. The upper back muscles attached to the scapula and shoulders keep your spine upright, stabilize your shoulder girdle, connect your arms to your torso and form the natural curves of your upper back. These muscles provide support for your upper spine just like your core muscles provide support for your trunk. They overlap and run in different directions to provide spinal stability and trunk mobility. You can feel this connection on your own by pulling your shoulder blades together. Do you feel your chest open? Now, move the opposite way to spread your shoulder blades open. If this is difficult, then you may have some upper back muscle weakness or tightness. This also amounts to a lack of scapula stabilization, or not being able to keep the shoulder girdle stable. Two common symptoms are: 1) the shoulder blades protruding or not resting flat on your back and 2) the shoulders lifting toward your ears. Both of these positions compromise shoulder stability and can eventually alter the natural curve of your upper back.

The trapezius muscles, or traps for short, form a diamond shape that runs from the base of your skull to the back part of your shoulders and then down to the middle of your back. This muscle is divided into upper or lower traps; it is often the upper traps that overwork, causing the shoulders to elevate, when the surrounding muscles are weak or imbalanced. In between your shoulders blades are the rhomboids, which protract or bring your shoulder blades closer together. To feel this connection, try bringing your shoulder blades together and then open them.

The serratus anterior is a small, thin stabilizing muscle that covers the lateral rib cage and connects to your shoulder blades; it holds your shoulder blades in place, assisting in shoulder stabilization. If your shoulder blades protrude, it is usually caused by weakness of this muscle. The biggest muscle of the back is the latissimus dorsi or lats, which wrap from your sacrum to your front ribs to provide spinal support. *It takes a combination of these muscles to help maintain the natural curves of the upper back.*

As you have read, a rounded back posture may be an indication of a series bone disease—osteoporosis. So take a very good look at your spine. Presuming that you don't have a bone disease, some imbalances can be corrected.

Shoulder Tightness Test

Shoulder tightness, for example, can be determined with this simple test. This is just one of many examples of tightness in your upper back.

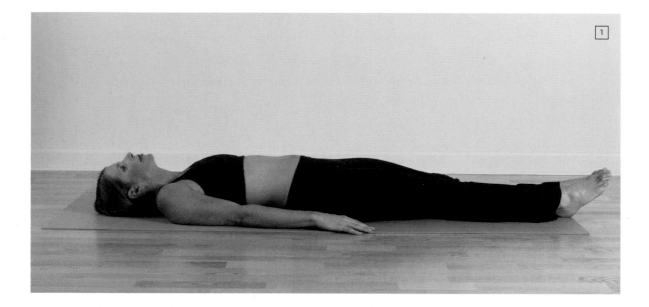

1

1 Lie on your back, with your legs extended and arms by your sides. If your chin juts to the ceiling, creating a severe arch in your neck, then that may indicate that you have tightness in your shoulders.

2 To balance the head, neck and shoulders, place a pad or folded towel under your head. Work with this towel under your head until you don't need it any longer.

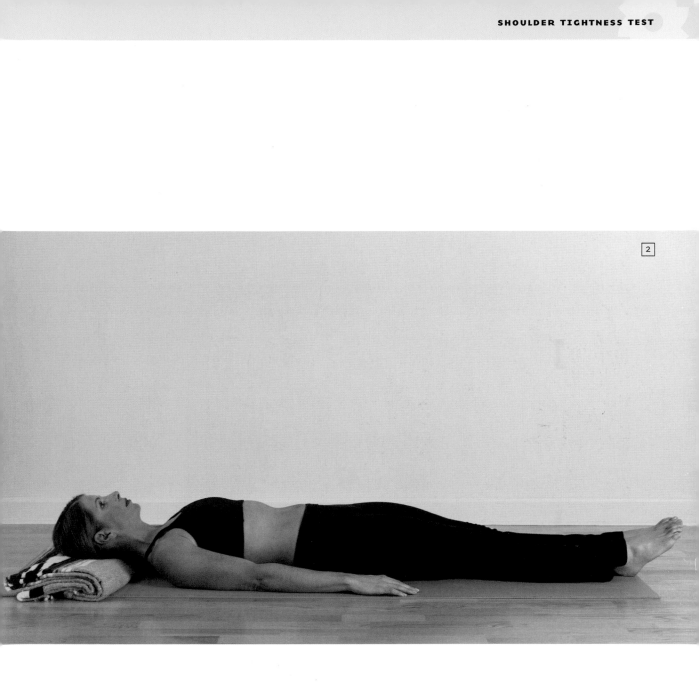

Stabilize Your Upper Trunk
by Drawing Your Shoulder Blades Down Your Back

These exercises will help strengthen and stretch the core as a whole, including your upper back, helping to relieve some of this tightness. While performing all of the exercises in this book (and during all movement and exercise), try to drop your shoulders toward your hips and keep your back in a neutral, slightly curved position. You can work toward shoulder blade stabilization by lifting your shoulder to your ears and then gently guiding them back so they can slide down your back. As you draw the shoulder blades in the direction of your hips, press from underneath your arm pits as well. Think of the movement as "Pits to your Hips."

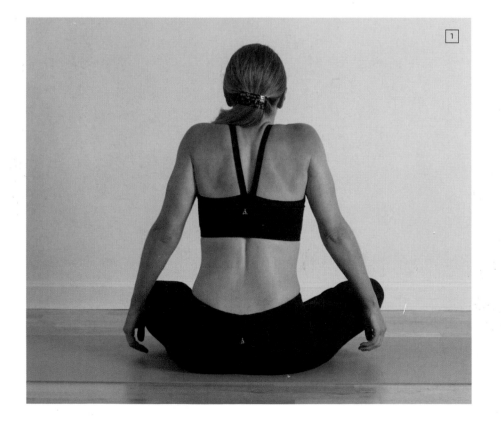

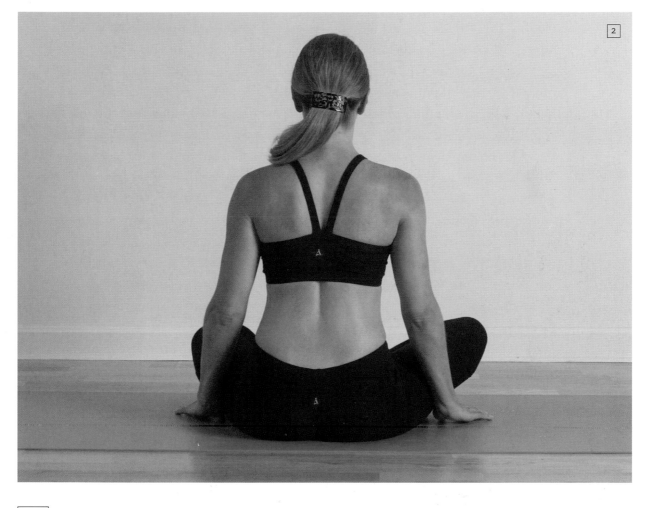

2

1   In a sitting position, draw your shoulders up to your ears.

2   Slide your shoulder blades down your back to strengthen the muscles that draw your armpits to your hips.

THE CHIN TO CHEST CONNECTION

If your neck and upper back feel tired and tense most days, then you probably can't just blame your boss or stress. You may hold your head wrong due to a combination of weakness and tightness. Any weakness in the neck can mean trouble for the rest of the body. When your neck and upper back muscles fatigue, then your heads tends to tilt forward, leading to neck stiffness, pain, and back problems. There are three major neck muscles. You have two primary muscle groups behind your head, the levator scapulae, which extend from just below the back of your skull and attach to your shoulder blades, and the upper trapezius muscle, which runs from the base of your skull past your shoulder blades. The levator scapulae lie on top of the upper trapezius muscles. Together, they tilt your head back and forth. On the front of your body is a thick, very visible muscle that tilts the head sideways and moves the chin to the chest—the sternocleidomastoid. In almost all of these exercises, you will direct your chin to your chest. Notice that this position creates length in the back of your neck. But here's a warning: If you have neck tension, then the muscles at the back of your neck may be short and tight, preventing you from bringing your chin to your chest or curling your chin to your chest. Forcing a tight neck to work is not a good idea. You can strain the ligaments and muscles, so don't force it. Rather, let the muscles stretch naturally at their own pace by placing a towel under your head as shown on page 67. Sometimes that is enough of a stretch. Begin by building neck strength with the mini-exercise on the next page.

Neck Strength Builder

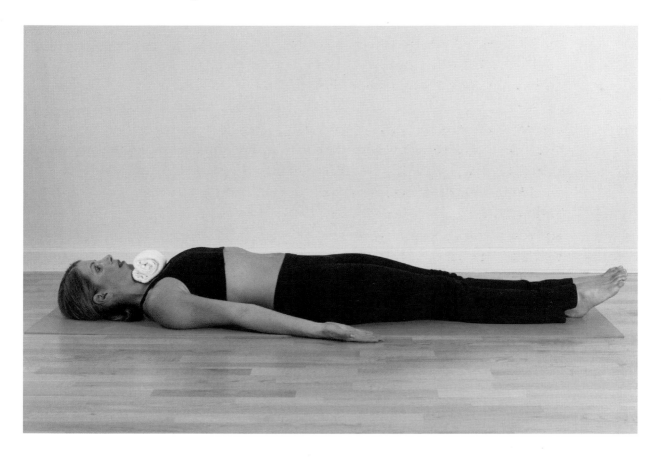

1 Lie on your back with your legs extended and your pelvis in neutral. Place a rolled up towel between your chin and chest—feel the length behind your head. Stop here if you can't draw your chin to your chest on your own.

(Neck Strength Builder, continued)

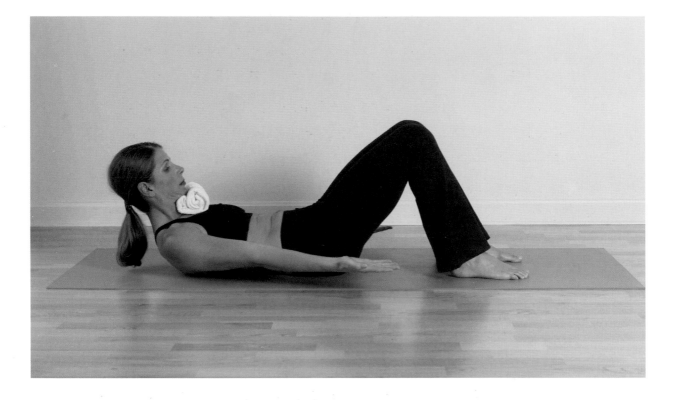

2 | Lie on your back with your knees bent and your arms extended by your side. Keep your palms up so you can feel the shoulder blades sliding down your back while the back of your shoulders touch the floor. Inhale to lift your chin to your chest, drawing your pits to your hips. Hold this contraction for five breaths. On each exhale sink the top ribs to the bottom ribs as if they are one—breastbone melts to the floor. Keep drawing your pits to your hips. If you need to, you can press the palm of your hands to the floor to help you hold the curl. After five breaths, roll back down on to the floor and rest.

HERE ARE THE BENEFITS OF A NEUTRAL SPINE:

- Neutral spine allows safe movements in exercise. If you exercise with your bones not in neutral, then you may not correctly train the muscles in the first place.

- Neutral spine improves overall posture by heightening postural awareness. The more you recognize the difference between good and bad posture, the easier it is for you to adjust your alignment on the job, at home, or in an exercise class.

- Neutral spine decreases the risk of injury. Doing exercises out of neutral can lead to injury. Maybe not now, but sooner or later bad form will result in the occasional twinge that can eventually escalate into chronic pain.

THE BREATH OF BALANCE

We all need to step back and take a deep breath from time to time. Oxygen is the most basic need for life, yet so many of us don't get enough of it. The entire respiratory system must work together smoothly and properly to give us the air we need. By definition, the respiratory system includes the nose, mouth, wind-pipe, the muscles that support the diaphragm, and all parts of the lungs. Your lungs sit in the body's chest cavity or rib cage, where they are protected. Basically, they work like to two balloons: Fill them up with air and then deflate them. As your lungs expand and deflate, they massage other internal organs and deep muscles, helping them work better, particularly the liver, heart and deep abdominals.

The real work, however, begins with two groups of muscles, the diaphragm and the internal and external intercostals. Upon inhalation, the intercostal muscles expand the rib cage, while exhalation retracts the rib cage, allowing the lungs to expand and contract. Your diaphragm is a thin, dome-shaped muscle sandwiched between the bottom of your lungs and the top of your abdomen that acts like a pump. As you inhale, it relaxes and moves downward creating a vacuum—sucking air into your lungs. When you exhale, the diaphragm expands into the chest to empty your lungs, simultaneously compressing your deep abdominals. *In essence, while working to allow you to breathe, the diaphragm also triggers a contraction in the deep abdominals. Your breath strengthens your core and protects your lower back from injury. The breath and body work in harmony.*

In a forced, or active exhale, you also send a message for your transverse and internal oblique muscles to tighten around the spine to protect it. You can literally feel this contraction—a belt or corset tightening around your waist. It's your breath that initiates this deep activation. If you don't forcibly exhale, then this process is compromised because the belly has a tendency to bulge, putting your lower back at risk for injury. Try it for yourself: Put your hands on your belly. Inhale through your nose, and then slowly let all the air out through your mouth as if you're frosting a very cold window with your breath. As you exhale deeper, draw your navel to your spine, creating a hollow abdomen. This is the position in which you need to hold your abdomen while doing these exercises, to protect your spine and avoid developing a bulging belly.

THE WORKHOUSE OF THE RESPIRATORY SYSTEM

The diaphragm triggers the deep abdominals by forcibly exhaling; you should feel this deep abdominal contraction as the muscles tighten like a belt around your waist. This, in turn, will protect your spine from injury as you build core strength. Your goal is to completely empty your lungs, exhaling deeply to trigger your transverse within every exercise.

After taking several breaths in and out, how do you feel? Relaxed? Calm? Peaceful? Your breath calms your mind as well. Breathing is essential to body awareness, core strength, and healthy exercise. Proper breathing keeps you centered in your workout. If you lose focus on your breath while doing these exercises, don't beat yourself up about it; simply bring your attention back to the breath as soon as you realize your concentration has lapsed.

If, during exercise, your breathing is restricted to the point where you're gasping for air, then just relax. Perhaps you've lost some flexibility in your diaphragm and intercostals, so they might not be operating at their optimal potential—not fully expanding. After all, if you don't use them, then they too will weaken just like any other muscle in your body. But, you will strengthen them as you progress through the exercises. Stress and tension are another story. They, too, can restrict your breathing. Remember an event that angered you. What happened to your breath? Was it shallow and labored? If so, more than likely, your breath had become constricted and restricted to your upper chest area, rather than using your entire chest cavity. You were probably not providing your body with enough oxygen, which only exasperates any tense emotional situation. By taking a few deep breaths, you could have calmed yourself down. Entire books have been devoted to the breath and its benefits. If you want more information on stress management, then pick one of them up. For now, remind yourself—take your deepest breath and exhale, exhale, exhale. Take your deepest breath and you will:

- ☉ Trigger your deep abdominal muscles to strengthen your core

- ☉ Strengthen the muscles of the respiratory system, particularly the intercostals and diaphragm

- ☉ Purify the body of the toxins lactic acid and carbon dioxide

- ☉ Release stress and tension. Deep breathing will relax you. At the same time, however, deep breathing may release emotions you have repressed. Their release may manifest as stress, tension, or negative emotions.

- ☉ Heal your body and mind by bringing more oxygen to the working organs

- ☉ Fuel every part of your body with precious nutrients; every cell within your body needs oxygen to optimally perform.

CORE CHECK UP

The mini-exercises presented in this chapter will help you to become more aware of your body and practice consciously, so you gradually align your body and break bad habits that cause tension and can lead to injury. To do these exercises safely, you must stabilize your body before any movement can occur. Easy enough—right? Not so fast. The learning curve is long, so feel free to do these mini-exercises over and over again. Take your time and ease into them; if, for example, you can't bring your chin to your chest, then don't force the issue. And that goes for any tightness in your body. Loosen up and breathe; your body knows what it needs to become balanced and healthy. Once again, the core concepts you will learn:

○ Put your pelvis in neutral: Stabilize your pelvis by contracting your abdominals; your pelvis must remain in neutral at all times—no tucking or arching.

○ Zip it up: Core strength begins between your legs. Zip your sexy jeans up by pulling the pubic bone to the navel and then the navel in and up under your rib cage.

○ Liberate your shoulders: Decompress your head, neckm and shoulders by lifting your shoulder blades to your ears and then move them slightly back to slide them down your back. The movement is pits to your hips.

○ Connect your chin to your chest: Gently draw your chin to your chest, but do not force it. The head is in line with the spine the whole time.

○ Train your transverse by way of your breath: Exhale deeply in every exercise to trigger your transverse.

WRAPPING IT UP: CORE SECRETS

○ Finding neutral spine is the first step to protecting your health.

○ You must always work with a neutral spine and a stable pelvis.

○ By honoring the natural curves of your spine, you can decrease the risk of injury because neutral spine puts the least amount of stress on your body.

○ Core strength begins with your transversus abdominis, affectionately known as the transverse; it is the deepest of all the abdominal muscles and its sole purpose is to form a deep girdle of support for your spine, providing spinal stability.

○ In every exercise, you will engage your transverse to create a "hollowing" of the abdominal cavity.

○ Pelvic floor activation works in harmony with the deep abdominals to create hip and spinal stabilization.

○ The intercostals and diaphragm trigger the contraction of the deep abdominals. The breath and body work in harmony to protect your lower back from injury and help strengthen the core muscles.

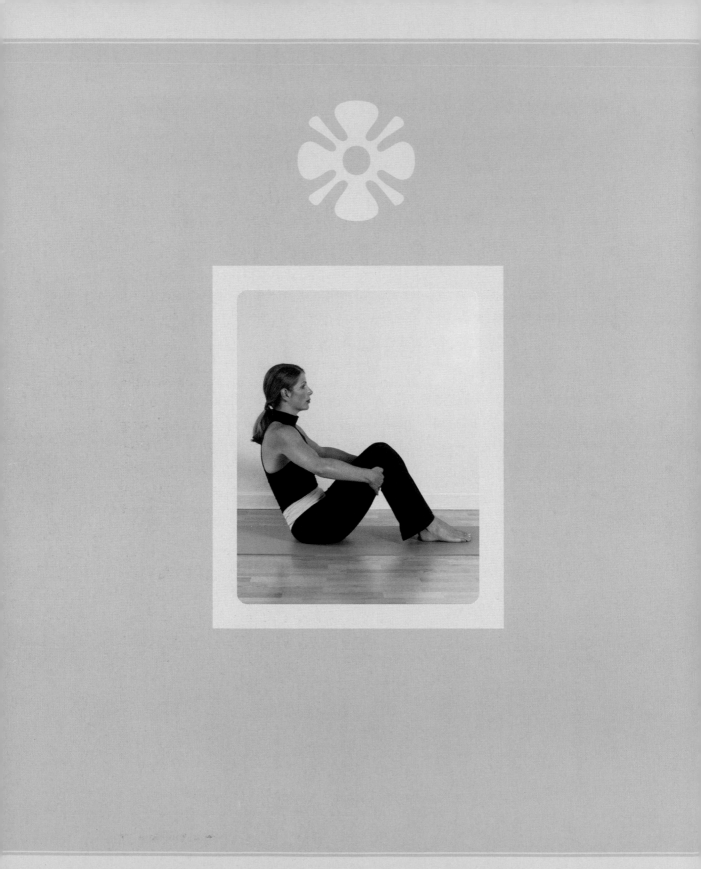

Chapter 4

Wake Up Your Core

The real challenge is getting started. This chapter kick-starts your training—waking up your core. After all, you probably have had little preparation for core work. Sorry, those crunches don't count!

To start, you not only need the physical ability to do the exercises, but also an attitude shift. Learning is process, a gradual evolution to a much bigger goal. Even in these starting stages, you will cover a lot of ground, connecting your breath to your body and your body to your breath. These beginning exercises ease you into activating your transverse, and your breath is at the center of this activation. Building real strength begins by feeling what's happening in your body and then gradually making the necessary changes. You may need to take more time stretching, for instance, so tightness doesn't block your core progress.

This journey is not a "get–fit faster" plan promising instant results. Any desire to be more advanced than you really are only sets you back. So, listen to your body. It is important to both feel the work in your body and to understand why you are doing a certain exercise. Don't overwork, making the fatal mistake that more is better. Rather, find a sense of accomplishment in just trying. Meanwhile, you are building a foundation for the body you want!

CORE EXERCISE BASICS

To make your core training complete, here are some more suggestions:

- Always begin with a cardio workout. Not only does the body warm up, but you are working toward a well-balanced workout routine that includes core training. For example, a walking program offers the same benefits as running without all the pounding; it's a great way to begin.

- Allow enough time for learning before progressing to more challenging exercises. These workouts progress in intensity and will test your balance and core strength. Don't try to rush ahead; you may set yourself back instead.

- Be sure to integrate your breathing with all the exercises and stretches.

- Always respect your weakest link, which may be your abdominals and your lower back.

- Always move in control. Haphazard, fast, and furious movements have no place in training the muscles of your trunk. Remember, the mind must ask the body to move.

- At first, focus on breaking bad health habits slowly—perhaps taking a few weeks to master one exercise and then move on. At the same time, try to add one good habit. If you try to incorporate every core concept at once, you are setting yourself up to fail.

- Begin every exercise by giving yourself a "Core Check Up": head, neck, shoulders, and pelvis.

- Invest in all the right stuff: a well padded mat, a fairly long belt, and a yoga block. Have a few hand towels around as well.

FORCING THE EXHALE

Your center consists of multiple layers of abdominal muscles that give your spine stability. Muscles such as rectus abdominus, internal oblique, external oblique and transversus abdominis form a deep girdle of support for your trunk. Triggering your transverse is the backbone of developing core strength. Your breath both centers your workout and activates your transverse. Exhale fully, force it if you have to, during every movement to activate the deep abdominals. This contraction scoops the pubic bone to the navel and continues as you exhale even deeper to hug the navel in and up under the rib cage. By linking awareness of your abdominals to your breath, you will also begin to feel how your body moves and reacts to each movement.

The Core Workout Exercises: Follow this program for four to six weeks before moving on to the next series of exercises:

Cat

Cat Cross Extension

Active Child's Pose

Active Hamstring Stretch

Supine Abdominal Series: Chin to Chest, Toe-Dips, Oblique Twist

Knees to Chest Stretch

Bottom Balance (modified)

Shoulder Bridge

Modified Spinal Extension Series: Spinal Push Ups, Push Up Extension

Active Child's Pose

Supine Spinal Twist (bent knee)

The Cat

BENEFITS

This exercise introduces you to core work, plus helps you develop shoulder and pelvis stability. Your goals are twofold, to lengthen and strengthen your core and to feel, by actually focusing on the tightening around your waist, the transverse contract. Cat also warms up the spine in preparation for the exercises to follow. Keep your breath flowing, with particular focus on the exhalation in which the belly button hugs to your spine.

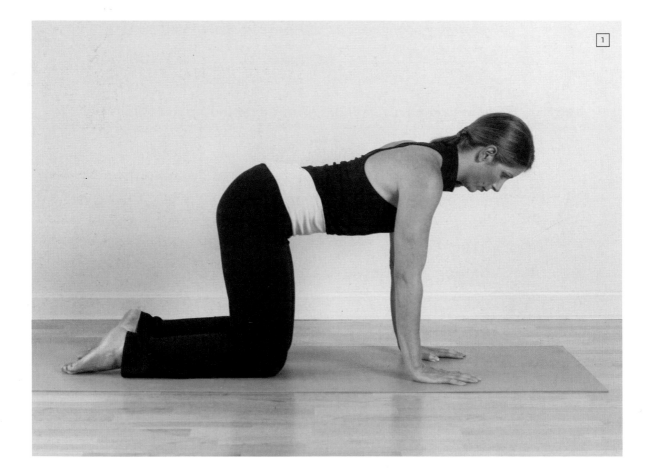

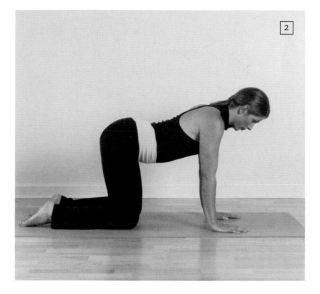

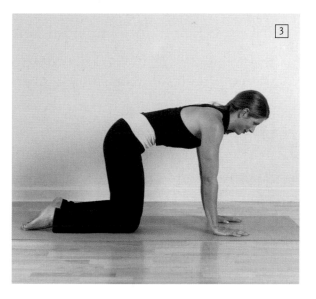

1 Place your hands and knees on the floor, your arms are directly under your shoulders and your knees directly under your hip bones. Activate your upper back muscles by sliding your shoulder blades down your back. Maintain a flat back and stable pelvis.

2 Inhale deeply, dropping your belly button to the floor. Your back may arch slightly.

3 Exhale deeply, hugging your belly button to your spine, lengthening from the top of your head to your tailbone. *Maintain a flat back, like a table top, even as the belly button pulls up to the spine. Use your breath to engage your core even deeper, hollowing the belly.*

Cat Cross Extension

BENEFITS

This exercise still focuses on transverse activation, only in a more challenging position to recruit more muscle fibers. Lifting your arms and legs off the floor challenges your balance and increases the workload of the core, buttocks, hamstrings and upper back muscles. This exercise also balances the muscles of the spine.

1   Place your hands and knees on the floor, your arms are directly under your shoulders and your knees are directly under your hip bones. Activate the upper back muscles by sliding your shoulder blades down your back. Maintain a flat back. Raise your right leg, lifting the heel of your foot to the ceiling, foot relaxed. *Hip bones remain even and pointed toward the floor, so you can maintain a neutral spine.* Then raise your left arm, palm down. *Focus on lengthening through the spine while hugging your abs to your spine. By pulling your belly button in and up under the rib cage, you can stabilize your body in this more advanced version of Cat.* Complete five full breaths in this position, and then reverse the leg and hand positions. Finish three to five repetitions.

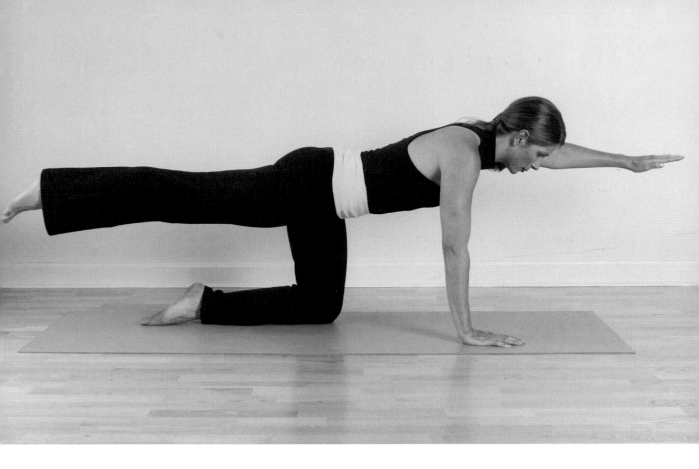

TRAINING TIPS

- Exhale deeper and deeper to trigger your deep abdominals and hollow your abdomen, navel to spine the whole time.

- Your waist shrinks with every exhale—imagine putting on your skinny jeans.

- Don't panic if you did not feel the transverse contracting. This action takes time, practice and some strength before feeling the "tightening" in your midsection.

Active Child's Pose

BENEFITS

Child's pose is a resting position to release tension, quiet your mind and nervous system, and stretch your back and hip muscles. In active child's pose you will also stretch your shoulders. You may recover in this position at any time and as many times as necessary. Your goal is to breathe naturally and relax.

1 From your hands and knees, open your legs so your knees create a "V." Open your heels with your toes touching, if you can. Slide your bottom to your heels. Leave your arms in front of your body, pointing your thumbs to the ceiling while your pinky fingers relax on the floor. Drop your head between your arms and then lengthen your arms away from your body to reap the benefits of the shoulder stretch. Breathe naturally.

TRAINING TIPS

- If you can't sit back on your heels, try widening your knees even more.

- If you can't rest your head between your arms, due to an injury or tightness in the shoulders, then place a block or rolled up towel under your forehead.

- Don't hold this position for more than ten minutes if you are not used to it; it may reduce the circulation in your legs, causing pins and needles or cramping in your legs or feet.

- Imagine sinking your spine and melting tight muscles away with your breath.

- If you have a knee injury, then you might skip this stretch.

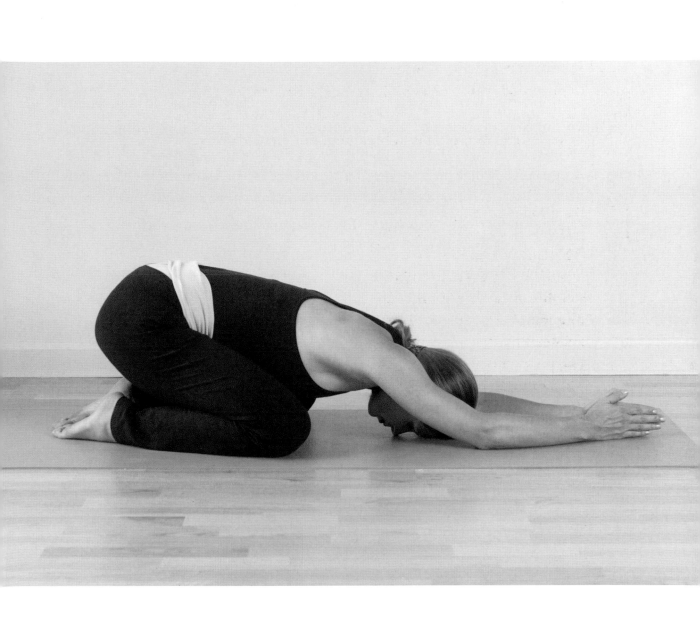

Active Hamstring Stretch

BENEFITS

This stretch focuses on the muscles of the hips, specifically the hamstrings, which run down the back of your legs. The hamstrings are a group of three muscles that have various roles in the body, but mainly they extend your hip and flex the knee. The *biceps femoris,* located on the outer back portion of the thigh, helps externally rotate the hips; whereas the *semitendinosis* and *semimembranosis* on the inner back thigh help internally rotate your hips. Most people neglect to stretch this area correctly, if at all. The problem is that tight hamstrings often drag down your life performance and alter your body appearance. Chronically tight hamstrings, for example, pull your pelvis down, locking it into a flat back posture. Poor posture, muscle instability, and chronic lower back pain are real possibilities. Whether desk-bound or enjoying morning climbs on the Stairmaster, you must correctly stretch the hamstrings as a group, not individually. Therefore, you will begin by stretching the center hamstring, then stretch the outer or deep abductor muscles (the outer hips), and finish with inner or adductors (deep groin). A good hamstring stretch is essential to creating length in your legs, improving your hip and joint mobility and reducing stiffness and pain in your lower back.

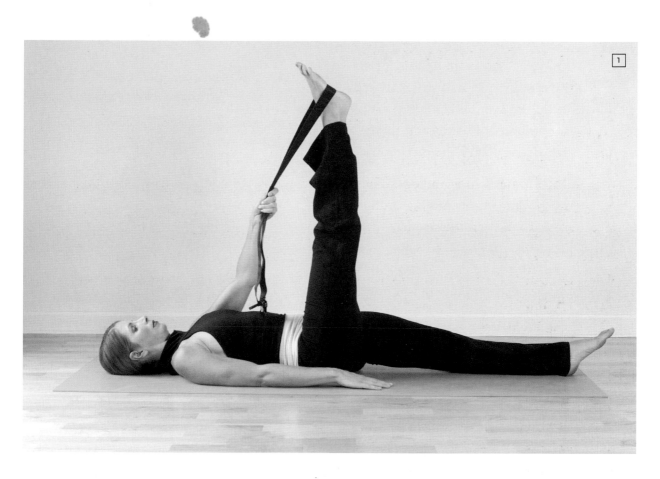

1 Lie flat on your back. Pull your right knee into your chest to wrap a towel, belt or rope around the ball of your foot. Extend your left leg, firmly pressing it into the floor. Inhale and slowly lift your right foot toward the ceiling, turning your toes out slightly. At the same time, press through the right heel to engage the stretch and gently push your left leg to the floor. Flexing your foot keeps the leg active to stretch the hip flexors.

If you want to deepen the hip flexor stretch, place the sole of your bottom foot against the wall, pressing the length of the leg into the floor. *Imagine your legs making the letter "L."* Hold the rope or belt with both hands as close to the foot as possible to deepen the stretch. Inhale to slightly release the rope; exhale to gently pull the rope bringing your toes toward your nose.

2 To modify your hamstring stretch, bend the bottom leg only. Complete ten to twenty breaths and then follow the rest of the directions.

3 Move the raised leg across your body while gently pulling on the rope to deepen the stretch. *You should feel the outer hip muscles stretching, which includes the outer hamstring.* Complete ten to twenty breaths.

4 Finally, move the raised leg away from your body. Keep the out-stretched bottom leg straight, toes flexed and active—do not let your hip roll in as your raised leg relaxes into the stretch. *You should feel this deep inner hip (groin) stretch, which includes the internal hamstring.* Complete ten to twenty breaths and then switch legs.

TRAINING TIPS

In this face-up position you may experience tightness in your shoulders and hamstrings.

- Shoulder tightness may prevent your head from resting flat on the floor. For example, your shoulders may elevate and your chin may lift toward the ceiling. If that's the case, then you are creating a severe arch in your neck, perhaps overstraining your cervical spine. Place a towel under your head to create a little lift (and comfort) and to help release and stretch your shoulders. Your chin should also draw closer to your chest. Words of warning: Don't work with an exaggerated arch in your neck; this position puts too much pressure on your neck. And don't force your chin to your chest. Use the props (review the Core Concepts in Chapter Three), allowing a few weeks for proper stretching to make it possible for your neck to reach this position easily.

- If you can't straighten your legs, then perhaps your hips are tight. Try bending your resting leg on the floor while maintaining the length in the raised leg. The goal is to gain in length, so try keeping your raised leg as straight as possible to get the maximum stretching benefits.

- If you have a hamstring or groin injury, proceed very cautiously, if at all.

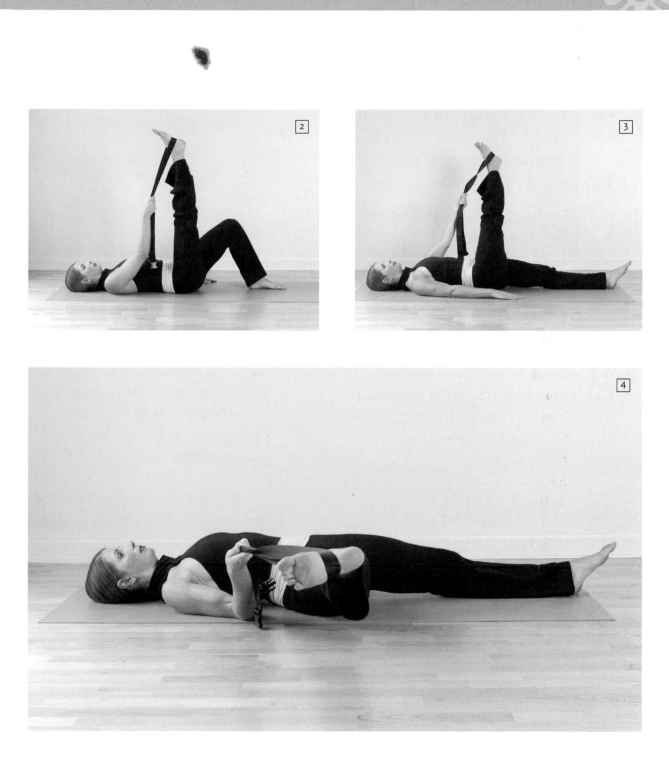

Supine Abdominal Series:
Chin to Chest, Toe-Dips, Oblique Twist

Chin to Chest

BENEFITS

This series of ab strengtheners targets your abdomen: transverse, internal and external oblique, and rectus. Strengthening the abs as a whole builds symmetry within your trunk and real core strength. Your goals are many: learning to curl up with good form, holding your chin to your chest to begin to develop abdominal and neck strength, and anchoring your navel to your spine, never lifting the lower back off the floor.

1 Lie on your back, drawing your knees to your bottom, feet flat. Interlace your fingers behind your head.

2 Bring your knees to a 90 degree angle—*knees in line with your hip bones*. As you anchor your lower back to the floor, gently interlace your fingers behind your head. Bring your chin to your chest, curling your torso up so the top of your shoulder blades lift off the floor, activating your abdominal muscles—direct your gaze between your thighs. Hold this position, and focus on your core. *As you breathe, sink the belly to the mat every time.* Complete five breaths in this position, focusing on pulling the belly button in and up under the rib cage on each exhale. Finish by lowering your head to the floor, but keep your knees in position.

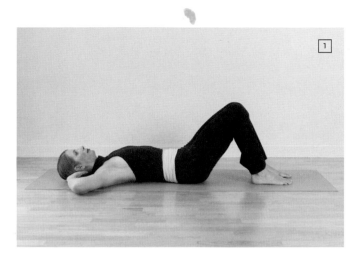

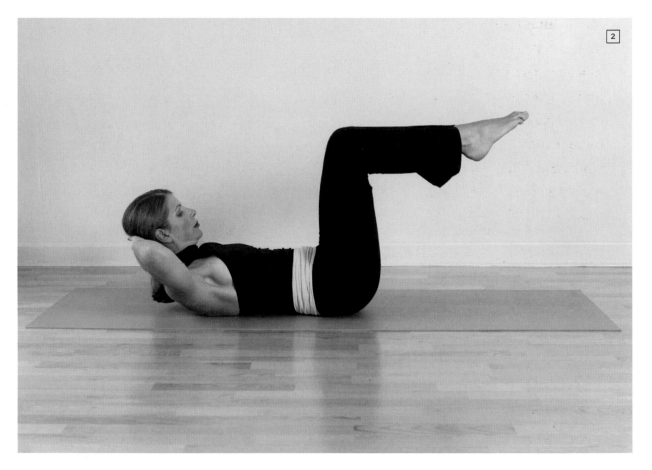

Toe-Dips

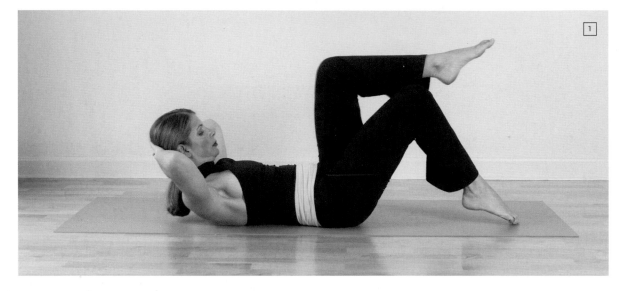

1 Lie on your back with your knees in a 90 degree angle. Gently interlace your fingers and place them behind your head. Curl your the chin to your chest, bringing the top of your shoulder blades off the floor, activating your abdominal muscles—gaze between your thighs. Focus on a neutral pelvis as you inhale to lower your right tocs slowly to the floor—*imagine dipping your toes into hot boiling water*—and then consciously exhale as you return your right leg to the starting position.

2 Inhale to lower your left toes to the floor and then forcefully exhale, returning your left leg to its starting place—you should feel your top ribs melting toward your bottom ribs, strengthening your abs, lengthening your back. Complete five sets.

3 In the same starting position, inhale to dip all ten toes to the floor and then fully exhale to lift your toes. Your pelvis remains in a neutral position as your legs move. Imagine your abs glued to your spine, creating core stability. Complete five sets.

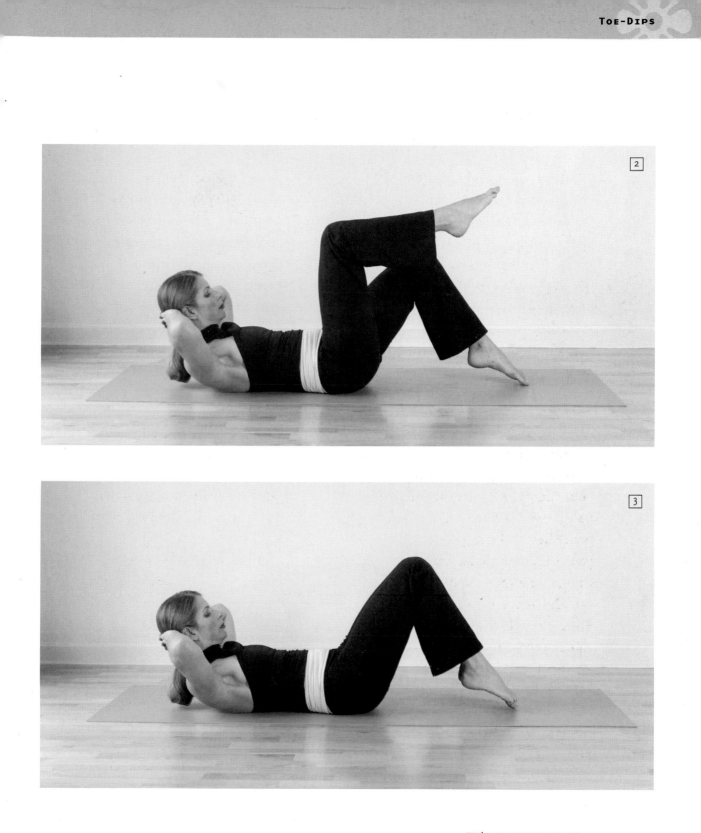

Oblique Twist

1 In the same starting position, inhale to prepare for the movement. Exhale and twist your left elbow past your right knee while lengthening your left leg. Hold this twist for three full breaths, sinking the belly deeper, twisting a little further with each breath. Return to the starting position.

2 Twist the right elbow to the left knee while lengthening your right leg. In this exercise, you are holding this contraction, deepening the contraction with each breath. Complete three to five sets on each side and then rest. If needed, you can lessen the intensity by lifting your straight leg to the ceiling.

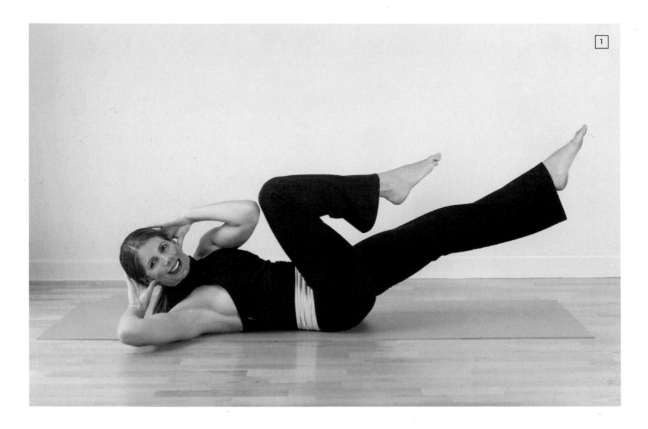

1

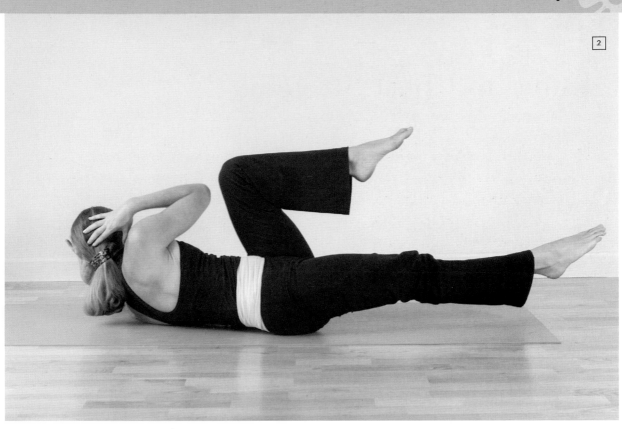

TRAINING TIPS

- If you get tired, rest. Good form is key. Less is always better if it allows you to maintain good form.

- Alternatively, if these exercises are too easy, focus so you can feel the tightening around your waist— completely exhaling and pulling the belly button to the spine every time.

- The goal is to keep a neutral pelvis while your legs challenge your core. Focus on your back—never lift it off the floor and don't bulge your belly.

- Do not jerk or bounce during the exercises. Always center yourself before moving on to the next exercise.

ARMS AND LEGS CLOSE TO CORE

Here's a tip. When starting out, keep your arms and legs close to your core. This way, you will not put too much pressure on your core muscles or strain your lower back. As your core gets stronger as a whole, you can then extend your arms and legs farther and farther away from your torso, progressively challenging your core.

Knees to Chest Stretch

BENEFITS

This stretch is a resting position that releases tension in your lower back, hamstrings and hip flexors, or psoas muscle. The psoas is the hardest working muscle in your body, mainly because it is responsible for lifting your knees to your chest. Tightness in the psoas, which actually weaves through your pelvis to attach your lower spine to your thigh bones, has lasting effects on your spine. When tight, it can alter the position of the pelvis causing an exaggerated arch in the lower back. You can rest in this position any time you want or need to.

1 Wrap your arms around your bent knees. With the strength of your arms, pull your knees toward your arm pits. Release the tension as your lower back melts into the floor with each breath. Imagine melting the bones of your spine into the floor; sinking your sacrum into the floor is the ultimate goal. Complete ten to twenty restful breaths.

TRAINING TIPS

- Don't let your back arch; allow no light underneath your spine.
- Check your neck. Don't let your neck arch or chin stick up. Put a towel underneath your head to create length behind your neck and shoulders.
- Melt one bone of the spine at a time into the floor—think of lengthening from the base of your spine to the top of your head.

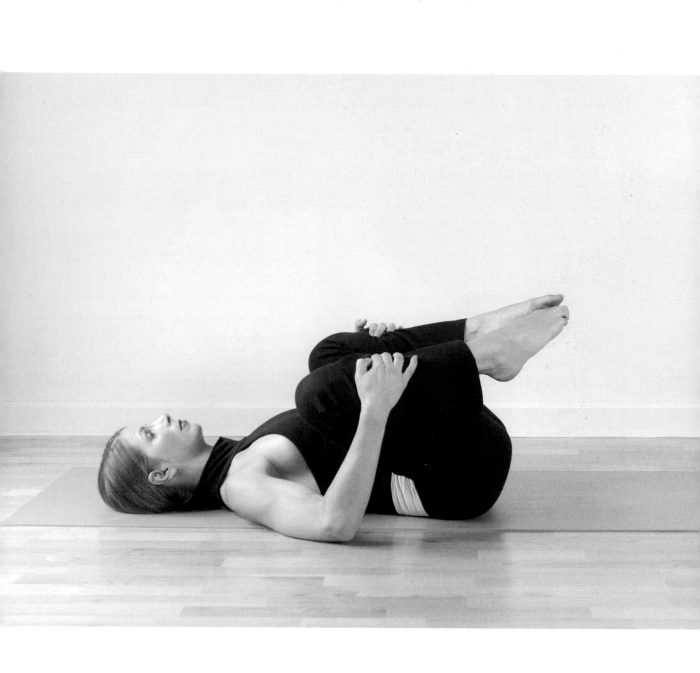

Bottom Balance

BENEFITS

This exercise targets the transverse plus prepares you for more challenging balancing exercises to come. Your goal is to make sure your belly moves the bones of your pelvis so it tips your pubic bone up and scoops your abs, creating a "hollow" abdomen; it's your breath working with your transverse that keeps your pelvis steady and you from wobbling.

1. Sit on your bottom with bent knees, grounding your feet on the floor about two or three inches away from your butt-bones. Place your hands on the back of your thighs.

2. Inhale to prepare for the movement. As you exhale, tip your pubic bone toward the ceiling and lift your toes off the floor. After you are in position, inhale and then exhale to deepen the contraction, pulling your pubic bone to the navel and then the navel in and up under the rib cage. Complete five breaths, then roll onto your back and pull your knees to your chest for a stretch.

TRAINING TIPS

- To keep the pelvis steady, exhale, exhale and exhale to fully activate the transverse.

- Imagine scooping out the letter "C" in your abdomen.

- Don't elevate your shoulders, even if you feel unstable. Try relaxing, sliding your shoulder blades down your back to engage your upper back muscles. This way, your core is completely engaged and active, creating stability.

- Remember, you are linking your breath to your spine to create balance, control, stability, and grace.

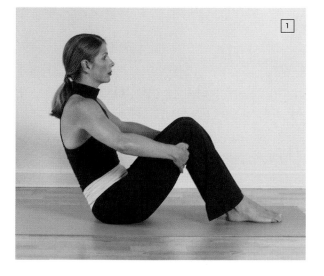

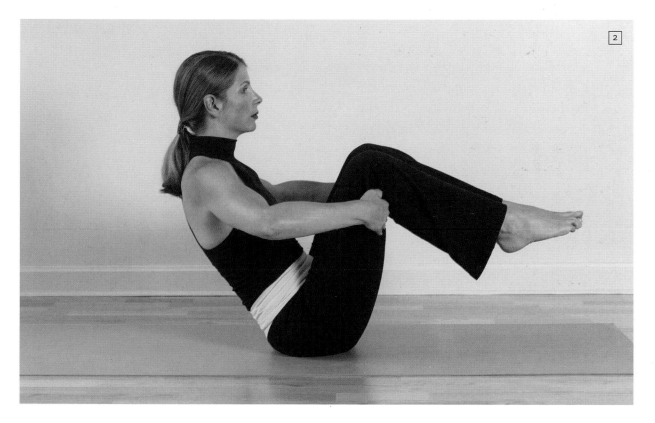

Shoulder Bridge

BENEFITS

This exercise strengthens your back muscles, hamstrings, buttocks, and inner thighs. At the same time, Shoulder Bridge stretches the quadriceps, psoas, and abdominal muscles.

1 Lie flat on your back with bent knees, with the soles of your feet on the floor. Lengthen your arms by your sides, palms down so you can gently press into the floor.

2 Inhale to prepare and press the palms of your hands into the floor, engaging your upper back muscles. Then exhale, tipping your pubic bone toward the ceiling so your torso lifts off the floor, peeling the spine off the floor one bone at a time—*imagine a string of pearls lifting one at a time off the floor, pearl by pearl or bone by bone.* After lifting your pelvis off the floor, lengthen your fingertips to your toes, so your body weight rests on your shoulders and upper back muscles, not your neck. While drawing your hamstrings closer to your bottom, keep your knees parallel and even. Complete ten to twenty breaths and then gently roll down, bone by bone.

TRAINING TIPS

- Focus on your knee alignment. Your knees should align directly over your heels. If your knees fall open past your feet, your thighs will tend to open too much. This misalignment lessens the inner thigh strength benefits. If, however, your feet are too close to your behind, this may cause knee discomfort.

- You should be able lift your head in this position. Don't put needless pressure on your neck; your upper back muscles should support your body weight.

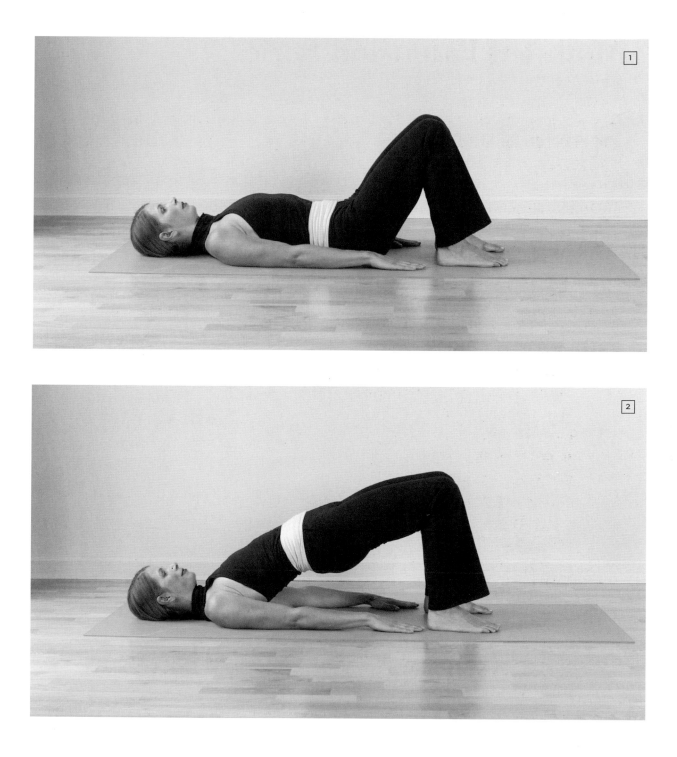

Modified Extension Series:
Spinal Push Ups, Push Up Extension

Spinal Push Ups

BENEFITS

After all of the curling up, you must turn your body the other way to work your back muscles and stretch your abs. Even though this extension is modified and targets strengthening the upper back muscles, it still works the muscles that run the length of your spine.

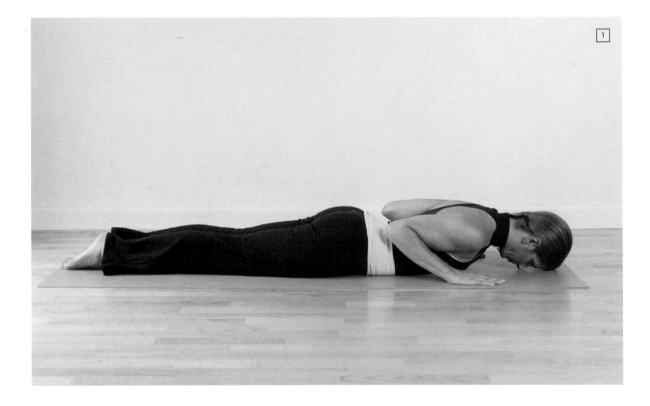

1 Lie on your stomach with your legs lengthened behind you. Place the palms of your hands directly under your shoulders, elbows pressing down to your toes and the floor. Gaze at the floor.

2 Inhale lifting the palms of your hands and chest off the floor. While lifted, slide your shoulder blades down your back to engage your upper back muscles. Complete three to five breaths. Rest. Repeat this exercise three times.

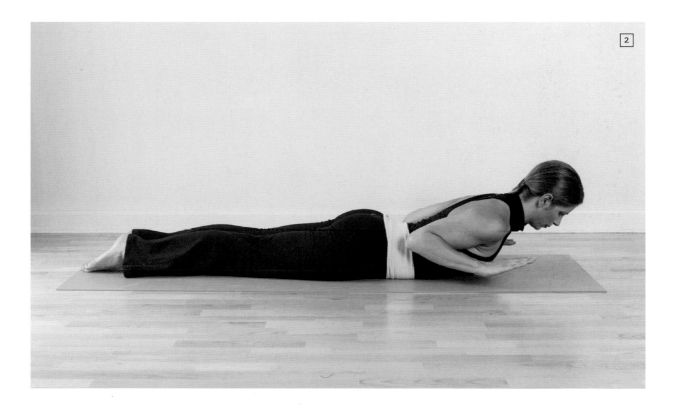

Push Up Extension

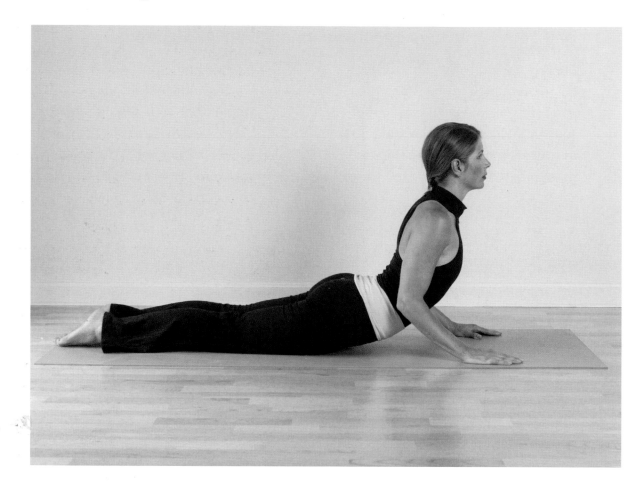

1 In the same starting position—on your stomach, with your hands directly under your shoulders—open your legs hip-width apart, still looking at the floor. This time, press your elbows toward the floor and then glue them to your rib cage. Inhale, pushing up into extension; it's the strength of your arms that lifts your chest and abdomen off the floor. *Imagine growing tall from the top of your head to create length in your spine.* Don't arch your lower back, rather elongate your spine. Complete five breaths and then return to resting position. Repeat three times and then relax in an Active Child's Pose.

TRAINING TIPS

- The most common problem is lack of scapula stability. The shoulders will almost always want to lift toward your ears, which is usually a sign of upper back weakness or tightness. Don't let them climb. Remember, press your elbows to the floor and glue them to your ribs. If you still can't control your shoulders, then don't push up. Remember, this exercise is an upper back strengthener. You can build strength slowly with the modified extension exercise. The important point is that you work with good form.

- To align your shoulders, press your elbows to the floor and glue them to your rib cage. This will prevent them from splaying out, which compromises your form.

- Draw your shoulder blades down your back to create scapula stabilization.

- Relax your buttocks so you don't over contract and push into your lower back; instead, lengthen from the top of your head, creating length in each bone of your spine.

- Extension of the mid and upper back is sometimes hard to feel without pushing or straining your lower back. Again, imagine growing taller and taller with each breath, opening your bones with your breath.

- Head positioning is also vital in extension. Do not look up at the ceiling; instead, gaze at the floor to create length from the top of your head as you lift, and then look straight ahead. Throwing your head back may strain your cervical spine.

Wake Up Your Core 107

Supine Spinal Twist

BENEFITS

This stretch loosens up your back muscles, which may be a little tender after the last few exercises, plus it cleanses your body and prepares you for a more advanced twist. Rotation is a natural movement of the spine and it keeps your spine healthy.

1 Lie on your back with your legs straight. Stretch your hands out to each side so your arms form a "T." Pull your left knee to your chest and then as you inhale, use your right hand to guide your knee to the right side of your body; it doesn't really matter if the straight leg rolls—just relax. Exhale and use your hand to gently pull your knee toward the floor for a deeper stretch. Look to the opposite shoulder. Complete ten to twenty breathes and then repeat on the opposite side.

2 Return to the starting position, and then pull your right knee to your chest and inhale to gently twist your knee to the left. Exhale deeper and deeper into the twist, while using your hand to guide your knee closer to the floor. Relax and smile—you're done!

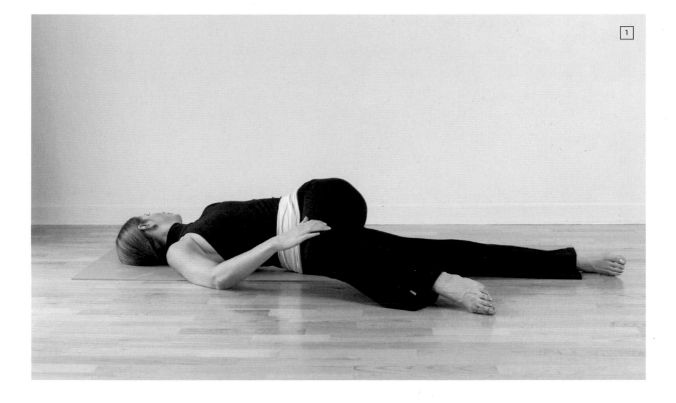

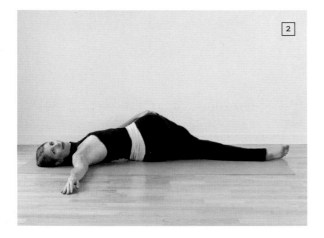

TRAINING TIPS

- If you have a spinal disc injury, don't do any twists. Please consult your doctor as well.

- Don't worry if your shoulders lift off the floor. Just relax and decompress after all the hard work.

PRACTICE IS PERFECTION

Congratulations! You have completed the first set of exercises. Take your time mastering them. Even if they seem easy, try focusing on your breath to create more of a challenge for yourself. Getting in touch with your transverse is crucial to advancing. As the intensity of these exercises increases, you should pay closer attention to your body. So, let's close this chapter by assessing what you have learned about your body:

⟡ Is there some type of physical or emotional limitation in your body?

⟡ Does one shoulder out-perform the other—higher or stronger?

⟡ Did you feel pressure in your lower back at any time? If so, did you exhale even deeper to create length in your back? Did this alleviate the low back strain? A little lower back soreness is not uncommon, but severe pain may be an indication that you have a serious back problem that may need professional attention.

⟡ What areas in your body were least flexible—the hamstrings, shoulders or hips?

⟡ Did you tense up when an exercise challenged you physically and emotionally?

⟡ Do you feel stronger?

⟡ Did you connect your breath to your body and your body to your breath?

⟡ Did you feel the transverse activation? Be honest!

WRAPPING IT UP: CORE SECRETS

- ✧ Keep your breath flowing through every exercise and stretch.

- ✧ Deeply exhale every time to get in touch with your transverse, as if tightening a belt around your waist.

- ✧ Even though your back remains flat, your abdomen "hollows" to work your core in unison.

- ✧ Move slowly and deliberately because every move requires your full concentration.

- ✧ As a general rule, work with your limbs close to your core to decrease the intensity of the work and reduce lower back strain. When your limbs work away from your core, the intensity of the exercise increases.

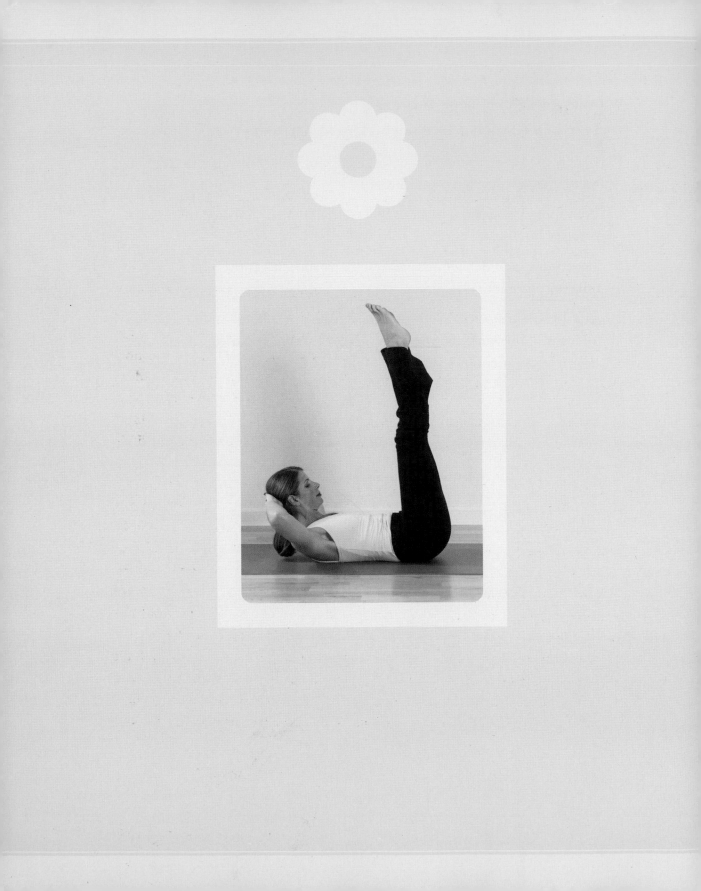

Chapter 5

Core Curves

Now that you have built a solid foundation, step it up a notch. Challenging your body with new exercises is only half the equation. The journey to self-knowledge is also essential to making over your body—and enhancing your life. Not only will you deepen your core connection with this next set of exercises, but you will also turn your practice inward to listen to the subtle, or not so subtle, clues springing from your body. If you listen, you will make real progress in your core work. Given that life's movements are often unexpected, these exercises will prepare you for life's twists, slips, and falls.

Much of what you do in this chapter integrates assorted muscle groups in a variety of positions, challenging your body from head to toe. Not only will you strike a balance between tightening your torso and building core strength, these exercises vary in strength, stability, and flexibility to prepare you for real life movement. You are building on the new-found strength of your muscles. They will be able to do more. And you'll be able to stretch and challenge yourself more, while learning more about your body. Self-study and self-observation are vital to training. These exercises are slow and controlled so you can better listen to your thoughts and your body's language. Perhaps you don't realize this, but your body spends a lot of time talking to you, in the form of a spasm, ache, twitch, or shooting pain. All are warning signs. An endless stream of negative thoughts also limits us in life and keeps us from having fun.

One of the goals for this chapter is to stay focused. You will still strive for a tighter tummy, strong back, and improved flexibility, but your real goal will be to strengthen your mind and muscles with careful attention to the messages they send you as you exercise. That will put you well along the path to self-mastery.

CHANNELING ENERGY UP

In the last chapter I talked a lot about the importance of engaging your transverse to strengthen your core and stabilize your spine. But there are other contractions that assist your core development. Lifting between your legs is one. Activating your pelvic floor muscles and contracting your deep abs help stabilize the pelvis. Think of it this way: Imagine a thick milk shake. You're thirsty, so you try to suck up the concoction through a thin straw, forcing your face cheeks to pucker as you suck harder and harder to draw up the milk shake in the straw. It's the same feeling! Only the contraction draws up through your inner thighs, groin and pelvis. You also want to engage your deep abdominals at the same time.

To feel this inward pull during the following exercises, work with a rolled towel between your legs whenever the exercise calls for it. One thing is for sure, deepening your core connection is difficult. So use the towel to help initiate the contraction, pulling the pubic bone to the navel, and then navel in and up under the rib cage.

PROPEL YOUR ENERGY UP

Deepening your core connection involves starting your muscle contraction from the root of your body—the pelvic floors. The pelvic floor muscles co-contract with the deep abdominals to create hip and spinal stabilization. Your pelvic floors consist of five deep layers of muscles that provide pelvis support, and prevent your organs from dropping to the floor. It is the hammock of the pelvis; the muscles weave through the bottom of the pelvis, from the pubic bone to the coccyx. Strengthening these muscles is not only necessary for core strength and general health, it's good for your sex life!

TAKING THE CORE CHALLENGE

Below is the list of intermediate exercises. Follow this sequence until you feel comfortable moving to the next level. If you do the entire series twice a week, you should be ready to move on to the advanced exercises in about four to six weeks.

Standing Core Activation

Wide Leg Shoulder Stretch

Abdominal Supine Series: Reach and Pull, Straight Leg Splits, Dead Bug, Straight Leg Oblique Twist

Knees to Chest Stretch (Chapter Four)

Modified Spinal Extension Series: Lift Arms, Lift Legs, Cross Extension

Active Child's Pose (Chapter Four)

Elbow Plank Series: Front Plank, Side Plank, Back Plank, Plank with Leg Extension

Hamstring and Psoas Stretch with Block

Spinal Twist (Bent Leg)

Butterfly Stretch

Standing Core Activation

BENEFITS

This breathing exercise helps deepen your core connection in a standing position. Since most day-to-day activities happen while standing, learning to activate your core in this position gets you ready for whatever your day throws your way. Remember, the goal is curving out a "C" from the pubic bone to the navel, exhaling so you feel the contraction of your pelvic floors between your legs. This breathing exercise also warms up your spine and centers your workout mentally and physically. Think about what you are about to do. Use your breath to clear your head and get you ready to build real core strength and stability.

TRAINING TIPS

- On every exhalation, you should feel your navel pulling back toward your spine. The added element is contracting between your thighs to create a deeper hollowing from your pubic bone to your navel and up, scooping a "C" in your belly.

- Remember the fundamentals of a neutral spine. First, your pelvis is neutral and must remain stable to fully activate your core and strengthen your abdominals. And second, your shoulder girdle needs to be stable: Draw your shoulder blades down your back to create a stable upper back.

- Use your breath to calm your mind and clear the clutter from your brain. The "to-do" list can wait. This time is for you, and for listening to your body.

QUICK TIPS TO FINDING NEUTRAL PELVIS

Tuck your chin to your chest. Relax your shoulders by sliding your shoulders blades into place. Place the palm of your hand between your pubic bone and thigh bone, moving your pelvis so your hand lies flat. Your knees should be soft and align approximately with your 3rd toe.

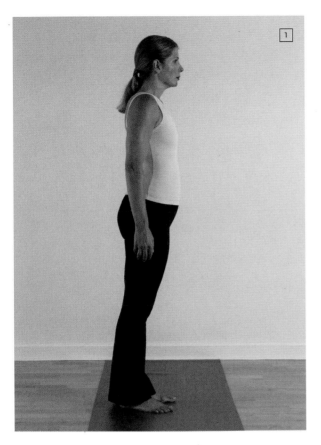

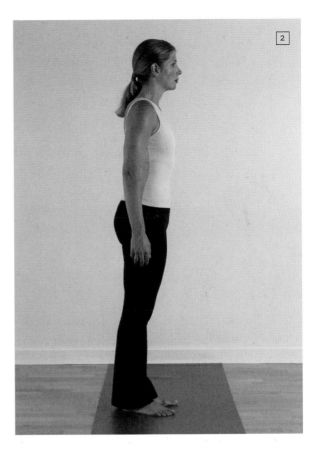

1 Stand with your heels together and toes slightly open. Lengthen your arms along your sides, drawing your shoulder blades down your back to prevent your shoulders from elevating. Place the towel between the upper portion of your thighs. *You must hold this towel in place so you feel the inner thighs connect to activate your pelvic floors.* Inhale for three counts, expanding your belly.

2 Exhale deeply, pulling your pubic bone to your navel and the navel in and up under your ribs. Complete five breath cycles: Inhaling for three counts, exhaling deeply for five counts. Eventually, you want to increase the length of the cycles to five-count inhalations and eight-count exhalations.

Balancing Standing Core Activation

BENEFITS

This exercise increases in intensity as you lift your leg. This is your first balance challenge. Your foot is the foundation for this exercise. Lateral stability will hinge upon the stability of the working muscles of your stationary leg, from your hips to your toes. Not only are you challenging your core, but all of the muscles in your legs.

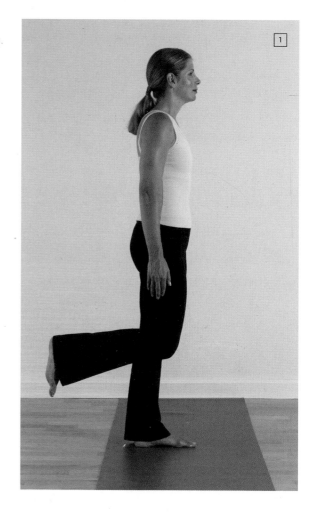

1   In a standing position, bend one knee until your shin is parallel to the floor. *If you are using the towel, hold it in place to feel the inner thigh connection and to activate your pelvic floors.* Complete five breath cycles: Inhale for three counts, exhale deeply for five counts. Repeat with the opposite leg.

TRAINING TIPS

- Try closing your eyes for the ultimate balance challenge.

- Ask yourself: How do I feel? What's happening in my body? Am I wobbly? Have I lost core control? Did the towel drop, even slightly?

Wide Leg Shoulder Stretch

BENEFITS

You probably never thought about it, but shoulder strength assists in any number of motions, from hoisting just about anything over your head to lugging whatever you carry during the day. These same overworked, yet delicate muscles need plenty of stretching. This stretch relieves upper body and shoulder tension. It also opens the hips and hamstrings. And, it is your first inversion, which helps to nourish your brain with fresh blood.

1 In a standing position, open your legs about 4 to 4 ½ feet apart, pointing your toes in slightly. Interlace your fingers behind your back, with the palms of your hands touching, if possible. Inhale to lift your chin and slightly arch your back. *You may feel a slight stretch across your chest.*

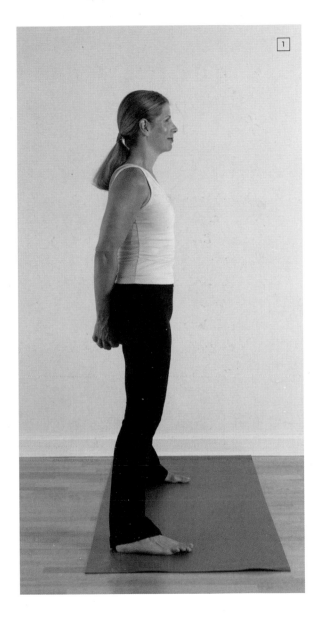

(Wide Leg Shoulder Stretch, continued)

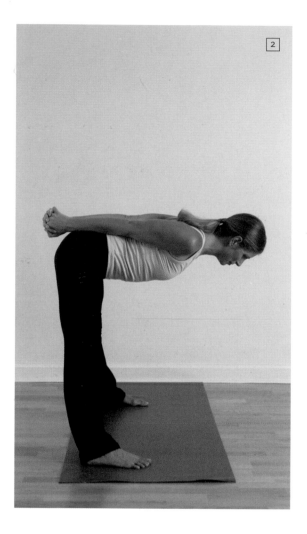

2 Exhale to bend forward from the hips, keeping your chin tucked to your chest.

3 Let your head dangle between your legs, lengthening the spine as you look toward your belly. Raise your arms over your head, palms touching. Eventually, your arms will reach toward the ground. Relax and complete ten to twenty breaths.

BODY TALK

Negative thoughts can lead to negative actions, possibly resulting in bad performance, even injury. Pain can sideline you, which begins a whole new cycle of negative thoughts. In order to heal your body, try to control your thoughts and turn your internal dialogue into positive affirmations. This is part of body awareness. Practicing emptying your mind during these exercises can also help make your workout a centering part of your day.

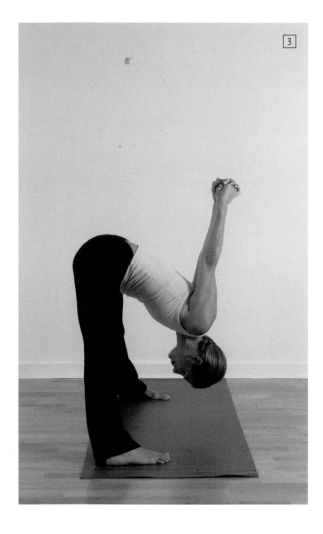

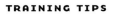

TRAINING TIPS

- Keep your arms as straight as possible with the palms connected.

- Relax your neck, jaw, and head. Tension has a way of locking up the face, especially the jaw muscles. Pay attention to these areas to melt the stress away.

- Keep your eyes on your belly, drawing your chin closer to your chest. You should feel a nice stretch across your spine, lengthening with every breath.

- In this mild inversion, focus on hugging your abs to the spine, despite their wanting to hang. Take this time to activate your transverse with every exhale.

- Engage your quadriceps, or thigh muscles, to lift your kneecaps to your hip bones so you don't lock or hyperextend your knees.

Supine Abdominal Series:

Reach and Pull, Straight Leg Splits (Isometrics), Dead Bug, Oblique Twist

BENEFITS

This selection of exercises integrates and strengthens all the layers of your abdominals. The goal is to glue the navel to the spine while your legs and arms challenge the abs. Because you will work with straight legs, the core challenge soars. But always anchor your spine to the floor; otherwise, you may feel lower back pressure. If you can't anchor your spine, try bending your knees or revisit the Abdominal Supine Series in Chapter Four.

1 Lie on your back with your legs straight out. Reach your arms overhead, stretching your fingertips behind you. Enjoy this stretch! Inhale to prepare.

2 Exhale and kick the right leg to the ceiling, simultaneously curling your torso so your arms reach for your straight right leg. Inhale to the starting position.

3 Exhale to kick the opposite toes to the ceiling, curling your torso so your fingers reach toward the straight leg. Inhale back down. Complete five sets and then prepare for straight leg splits.

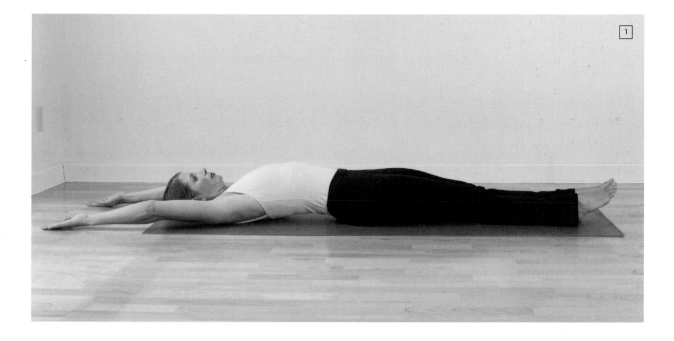

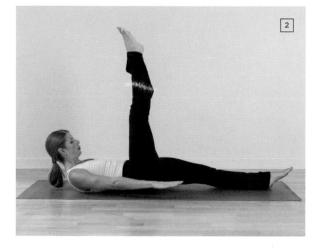

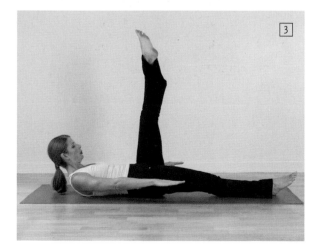

Straight Leg Splits

(Isometrics)

1 Lie on your back with your heels reaching toward the ceiling. Interlace your hands behind your head and curl your chin toward your chest, lifting your shoulder blades off the floor.

2 Drop your right leg, holding it an inch or two off the floor. The idea is to hold your leg in place while breathing deeply to challenge your abdominals in an isometric contraction (no movement). Complete five deep breaths and then scissor your legs.

3 The opposite leg drops to the floor; hold it an inch or two off the floor. As the leg lengthens, contract from your glutes and activate your inner thighs—*imagine that your thighs are pulled together by a magnetic force.* Finish five sets and then get ready for Dead Bug.

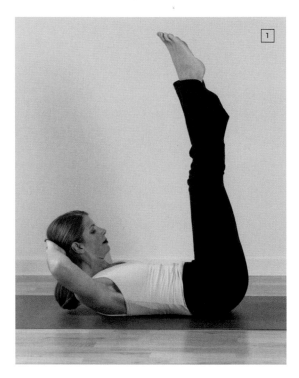

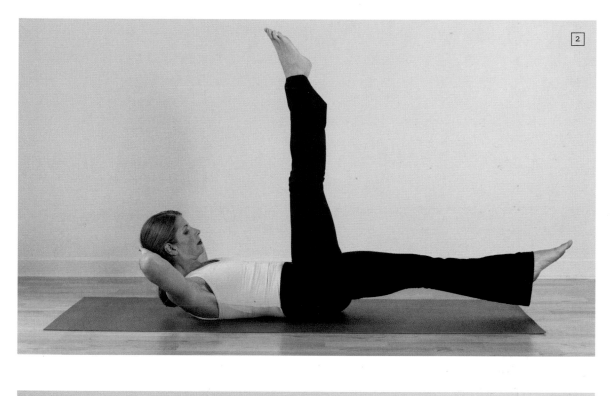

2

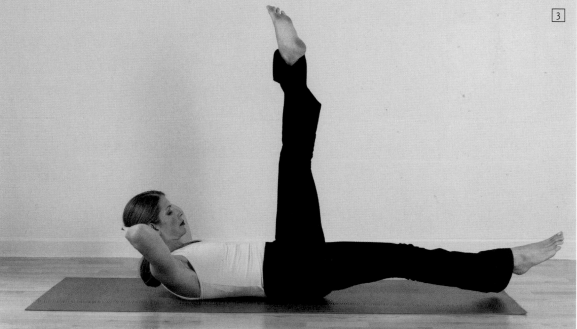

3

Dead Bug

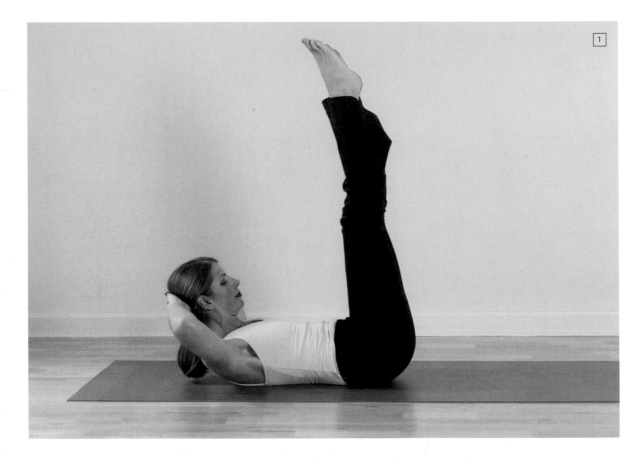

1   Lie on your back with your heels reaching toward the ceiling. Interlace your hands behind your head and curl your chin to your chest, lifting your shoulder blades off the floor.

2   Slowly inhale and lower your legs so your toes are in line with your nose. Then, exhale and reach your arms out behind you to expose your torso. Complete five full breaths in this position, exhaling so deeply the abs hug to the spine and then finish this series with Oblique Twist.

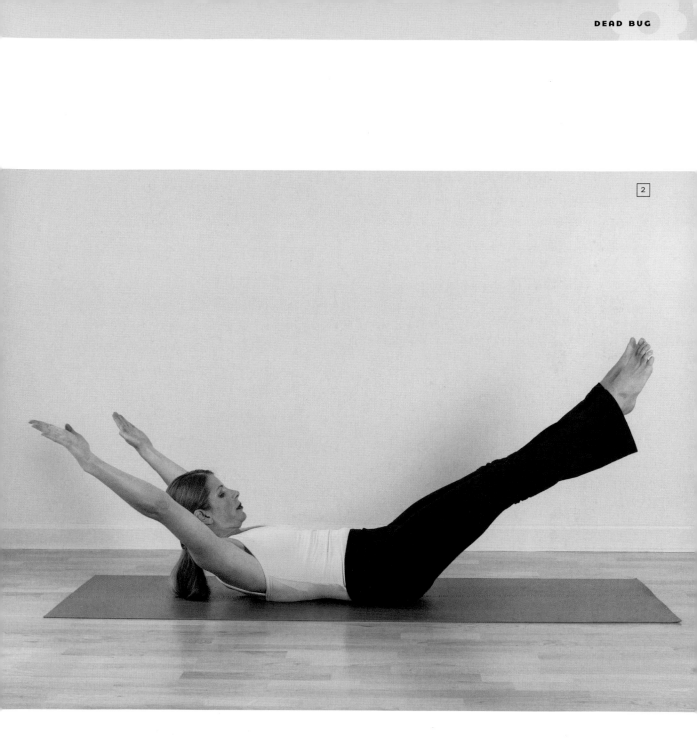

Oblique Twist (Straight Leg)

1 Lie on your back with your heels reaching toward the ceiling. Interlace your fingers and place them behind your head and curl your chin to your chest, lifting your shoulder blades off the floor.

2 Split your legs: The left leg lengthens to the wall, holding an inch or two off the floor, and the right leg reaches long to the ceiling. Twist your left elbow past your right knee and hold this contraction. Breathe deeply and try to extend your elbow past your knee with every breath, then scissor your legs.

3 The opposite (right) leg extends an inch or so off the ground. Twist your right elbow past your left knee and hold the contraction. Complete five full breaths, sinking the belly deeper with each breath, and then repeat with the opposite leg. Finish five complete sets.

TRAINING TIPS

- If you want to put a towel between your legs during the Dead Bug, then do so. You will definitely feel the pelvic floors contract, which helps anchor your spine to the floor as well.

- Remain perfectly still in your torso (except when the exercise requires a controlled rotation), even as your legs and arms lengthen away from the core. The idea is to challenge core stability and build strength.

- If you can't keep your torso anchored or your pelvis stable, then bend your knees. You can still get the same benefits at a lower level of intensity by bending your knees. Again, don't rush the core process. Core strength will come at its own, gradual pace.

- Maintain your neutral pelvis at all times. Do not arch your lower back. Keep melting your abs toward your spine.

- If you have or had a neck problem, leave these exercises out. The arms behind your head may put to much pressure on your neck.

- After you complete these exercises, stretch by pulling your knees to your chest.

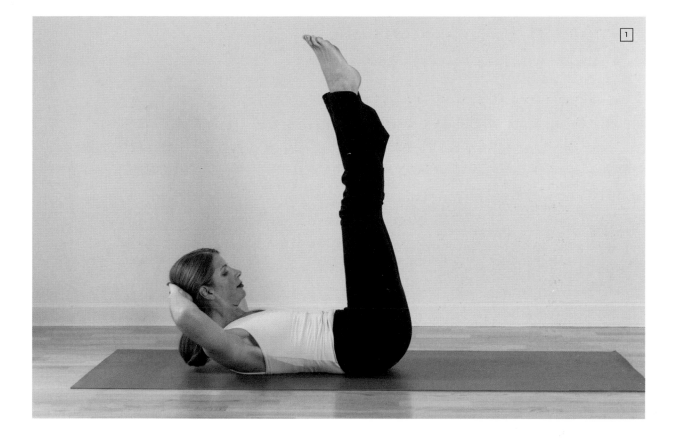

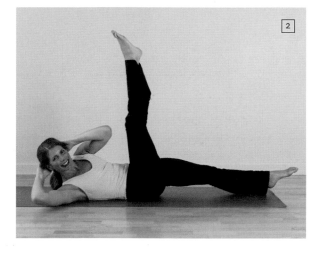

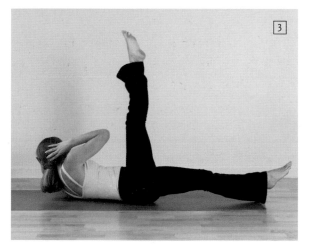

Spinal Extension

Lift Arms, Lift Legs, Cross Extension

BENEFITS

These variations of spinal extension begin to build a strong and capable spine. By strengthening your back muscles, you are also protecting your back against potential aches, pains, and injury. As these extensions increase in intensity, so does the workload for your back muscles. Not only will you strengthen the muscles running the length of your spine, but other muscles as well, including your hamstrings and the muscles of your buttocks. It's not uncommon to feel a slight stretch across your chest and the front of your shoulders as well.

1 Lie on your stomach with your legs lengthened behind your. Rest your arms on the floor above your head, palms down pressing into the floor to activate the upper back muscles.

TRAINING TIPS

• If you feel pressure in your lower back, try growing taller from the top of your head, creating length between your spinal bones.

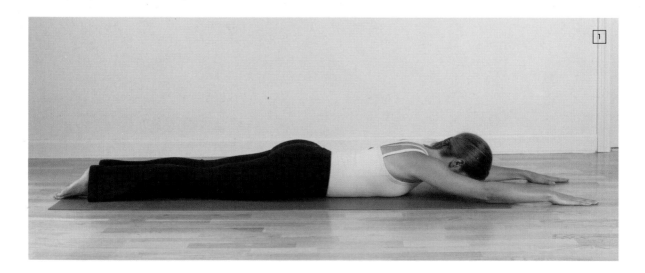

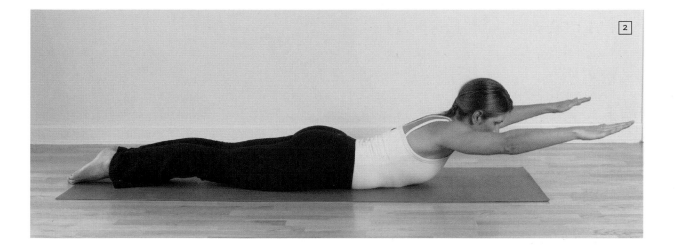

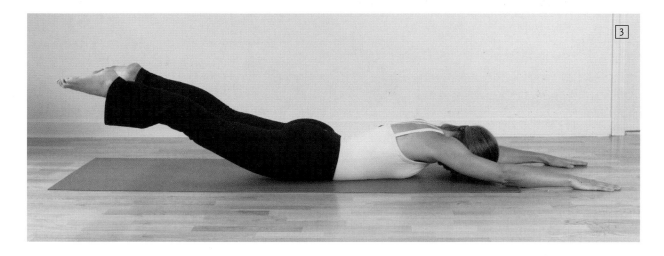

2 As you inhale, lift your arms off the floor—continuing the motion, peel your chest, shoulders and head off the floor as well. Imagine growing tall from the top of your head to create length in the spine. *Gaze at the floor.* Complete five breaths and then return to resting position. Repeat three times.

3 Beginning from the same preparatory position, lift your legs off the floor while the upper back relaxes. Lengthen your legs as much as possible to prevent pushing into your lower back. Stay active in your glutes and your core!

Cross Extension

BENEFITS

This exercise increases the intensity by targeting the back muscles in unison with the buttocks and hamstrings, while simultaneously bringing balance and stability to your spine.

1 Lie on your stomach with your legs lengthened behind you and your arms overhead, palms pressing down into the floor to activate the upper back muscles.

2 While you inhale, lift your right arm, lengthening through your fingers while the left palm presses into the floor. Next, while holding your arm steady and extended, exhale and lift your left leg while pressing the right foot into the floor. Hold for five full breaths and then switch sides. Rest in an Active Child's Pose.

TRAINING TIPS

- When pressing the palm of your hands into the floor, *imagine hanging on for your life as you sink deeper and deeper in a pit of quicksand. The goal is to draw your shoulder blades down your back, engaging your upper back muscles.*

- Think of lengthening from the ends of your fingertips to your toes.

- As your bottom lifts your legs, contract your glutes to sculpt your behind and, of course, stabilize your leg.

- Gaze at the floor so you don't strain your neck.

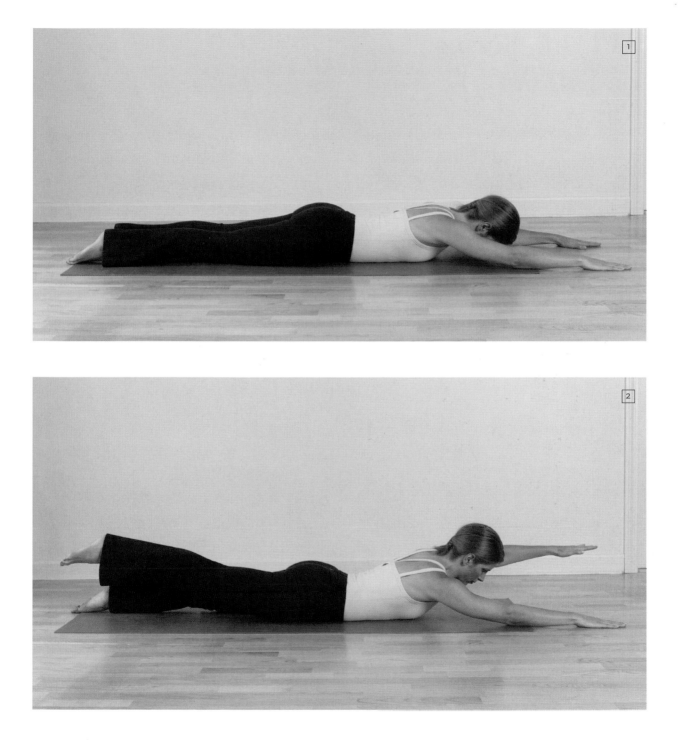

Plank Series:

Front Plank, Side Plank, Back Plank, Plank with Leg Extension

BENEFITS

The Plank is the classic waist trimmer; it strengthens your abdominals against gravity plus challenges your body in an integrated way. This means just about every muscle in your body will work to keep you stable—your abs, back, bottom, legs, shoulders, and pelvis. Place a rolled up towel or block between the upper portion of your thighs to activate the pelvic floors—you might need the extra help.

1 Place your knees and elbows on the floor. Your knees should be about a foot behind your hips. Align your elbows so they are directly under your shoulders, pinky down and knuckles touching. Gaze at the floor. With your toes curled under, place your heels together. Stay on your knees until you are ready to lift. Secure a towel between your thighs to feel the inner thigh connection.

2 Inhale and lift your legs, pelvis, and torso off the floor in one motion. Exhale and pull your navel to your spine while balancing on your toes and elbows—your body should be strong like steel, from head to heel. Complete five breaths. Rest and then repeat three to five times. Rest in an Active Child's Pose before continuing on to the Side Plank.

TRAINING TIPS

- Hold your core solid at all times or else your navel may sag to the floor. A sagging core shifts your low back into a severe arch, putting too much pressure on your lumbar spine.

- Pull your belly button to your spine at all times while squeezing the rolled up towel, activating your pelvic floors and inner thigh muscles.

- By sending energy through your heels, you can evenly displace your body weight between your heels, legs, core, and shoulders to help distribute your weight.

- Lift the back of your thighs to the sky, engaging your gluteals—maximize your maximus!

- Relax your shoulders away from your ears.

- And finally, gaze at the floor and lengthen the back of your neck.

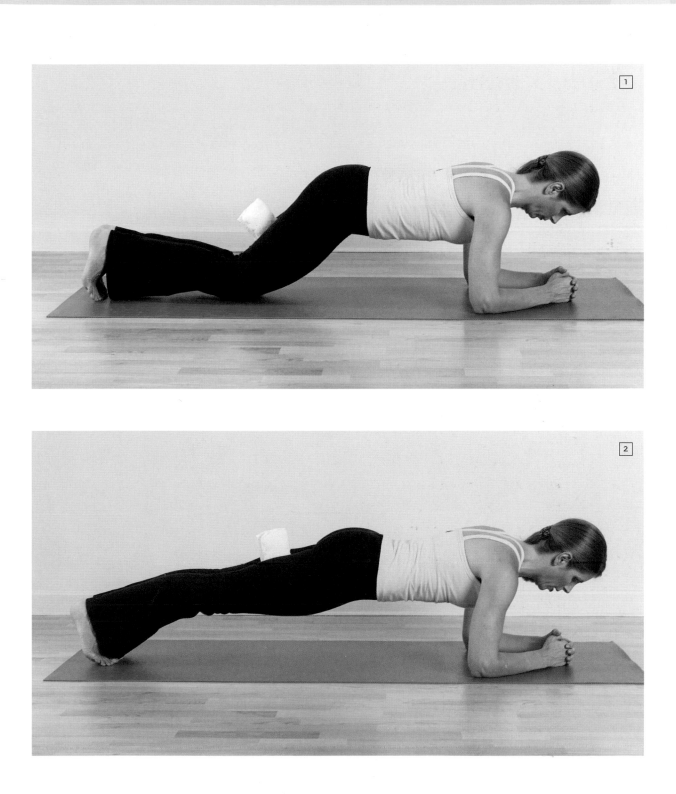

Side Plank

1 Sit on your left side with your knees slightly pulled into your body, stacking your knees on top of one another. Place your elbow on the floor directly under your shoulder. The towel is still between your legs.

2 Lift your torso, hips and legs off the floor in one motion. Balance on your elbow and the side of your knee. Rest your free arm on the side of your body. Complete five breaths and then repeat three to five times.

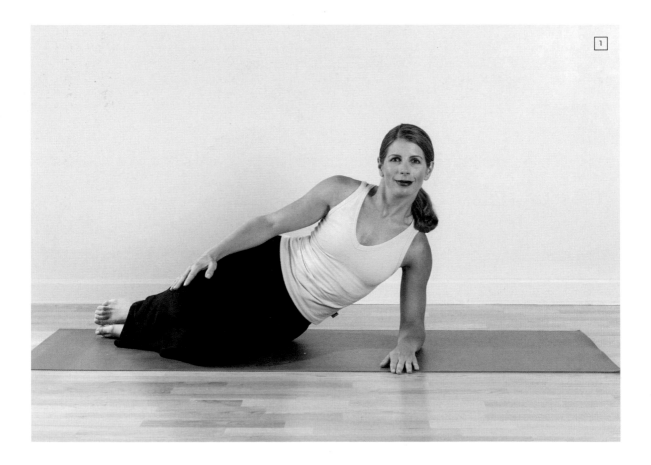

1

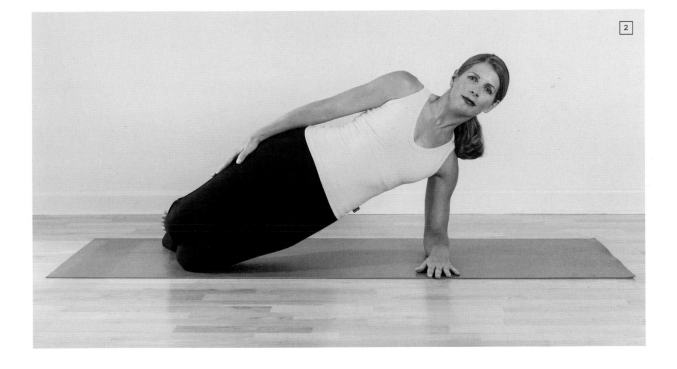

TRAINING TIPS

- Tighten your trunk. No drooping in the middle.

- Make sure your elbow is in line with your shoulder.

- Draw your shoulder blades down your back to prevent your shoulders from elevating. Securing your shoulder blades creates stability for your torso.

- Squeeze the towel between your legs to turn your pelvic floors on.

Back Plank

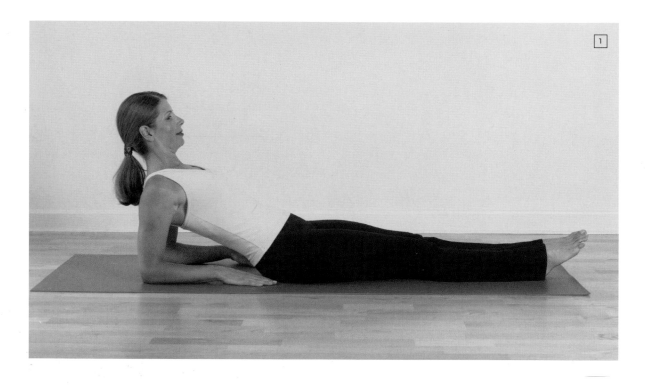

| 1 | Sit on the floor, legs straight in front of you. Prop yourself on your elbows so your elbows are directly under your shoulders, fingertips face your bottom. You may feel a slight stretch across the chest. |

| 2 | Inhale and lift your hips, bottom, and chest to the ceiling in one movement. Balance on your heels and elbows while gazing at the floor. *Point your toes to the floor to prevent any stress in your knees.* Complete five breaths and then repeat three to five times. Finish off this series with the Side Plank on the opposite side. If you still have enough energy, take it up a notch… |

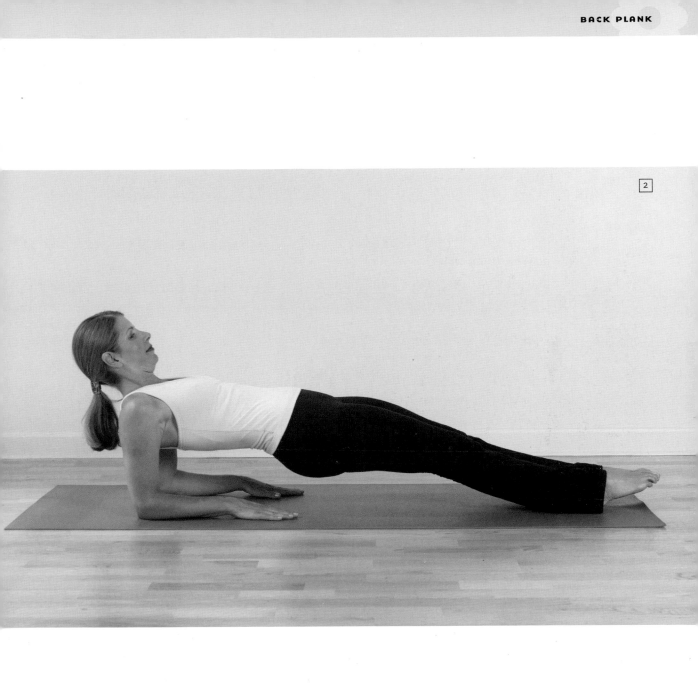

Plank with Leg Extension

1 Place your knees and elbows on the floor. Align your elbows directly under your shoulders, pinky down and knuckles touching. With your toes curled under, place your heels together. Stay on your knees until you are ready to lift into a plank.

2 Inhale, lifting your legs, pelvis, and torso off the floor in one motion. Exhale to lift the right leg, while balancing on your toes and elbows—*engage your behind as much as you can while lifting up from the core.* Complete five full breaths and then return to a plank position to lift the opposite leg.

3 While in the plank, lift your left leg. Complete five full breaths and then rest in an Active Child's Pose.

TRAINING TIPS

- If you have a shoulder injury, then don't try these Planks.

- Maintain an active, strong body and solid core.

- Always lift through the center of your body, keeping your inner thighs together to activate your pelvic floors which assist in stabilizing your body.

- If needed, rest in an Active Child's Pose any time during these Planks.

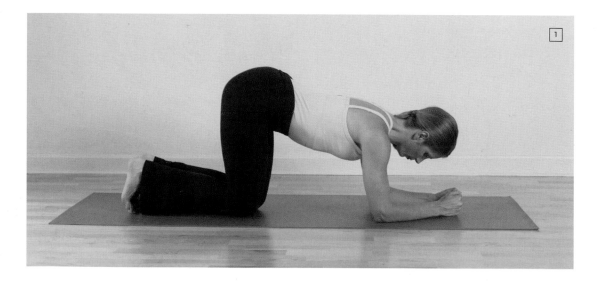

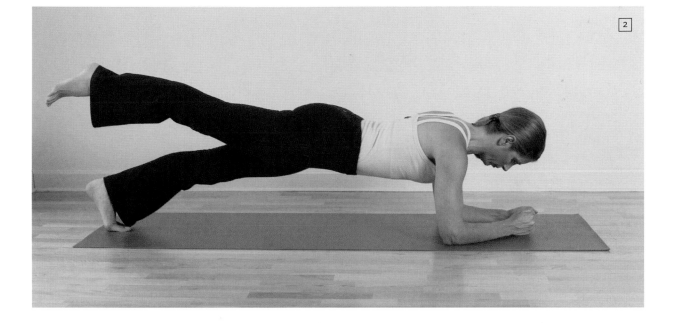

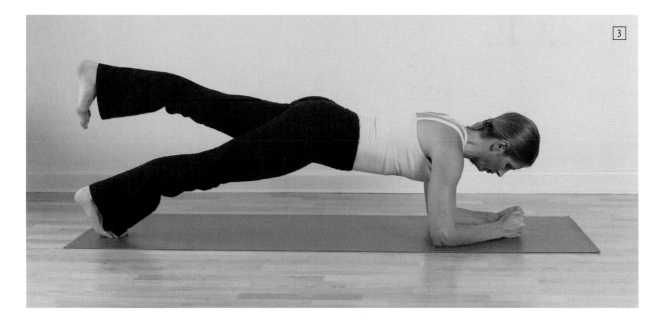

Hamstring and Psoas Stretch

BENEFITS

This stretch opens the back and the front of your legs at the same time. While stretching your hamstrings, you also stretch your groin, hip flexors, and quadriceps. Your breath, of course, helps relax your muscles so you get the maximum stretching benefits. You can try using a yoga block to ease you into this stretch, but it's not necessary.

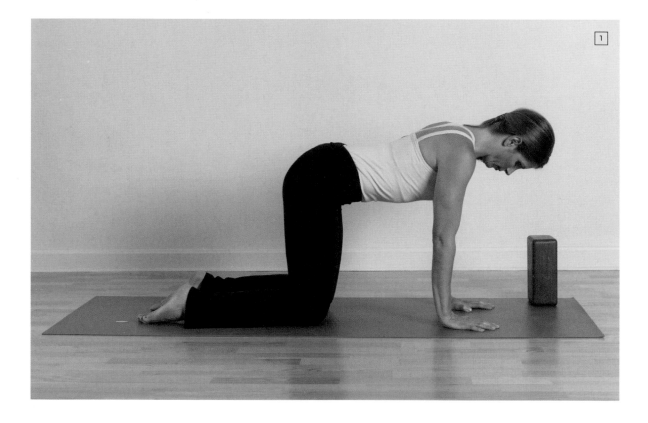

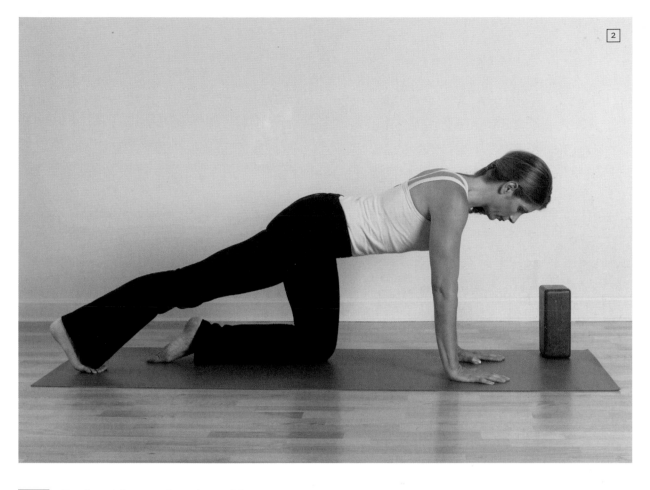

1. Begin with your hands and knees on the floor with your back flat like a table top. Have your block within reach.

2. Straighten your right leg behind you, curling your toes under.

(Hamstring and Psoas Stretch, continued)

3 Step your left foot into a lunge—your knee should line up directly over your heel. Your right leg stabilizes you. Your right shinbone rests on the floor; your toes can face down. As you fully straighten your right leg, press the thighbone to the floor, until your kneecap faces the floor. Don't rest your body weight on the top of the kneecap but on the meaty portion of your thigh.

4 Slide the block, depending on your flexibility, in a vertical or horizontal position under your left thigh. Use your hands on the floor for support, either on closed fists or open palms. Position your pelvis so that it rests in a neutral position, with both thigh bones facing front. Try to lengthen the back leg as much as you can.

5 Place your hands on your thighs. Complete twenty to thirty breaths and then switch legs.

TRAINING TIPS

- If you have a knee injury, then pass on this stretch.

- Make sure your body weight does not bear down on the top of your kneecap. Displace your body weight so it rests on the top portion of the thigh.

- You must maintain your pelvis in a stable and neutral position. Don't twist or shift your pelvis to deepen the stretch; this only reinforces poor alignment and stretches the muscles incorrectly. Both hip bones should face front and remain even.

- Don't rush setting up. Take as long as you need to get into the stretch—and moving out of the stretch.

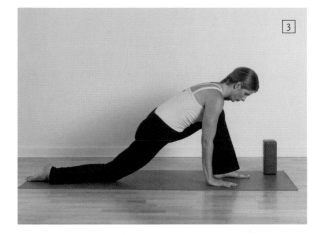

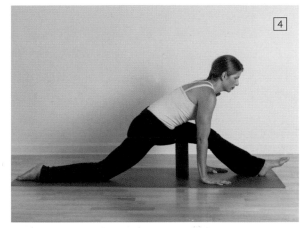

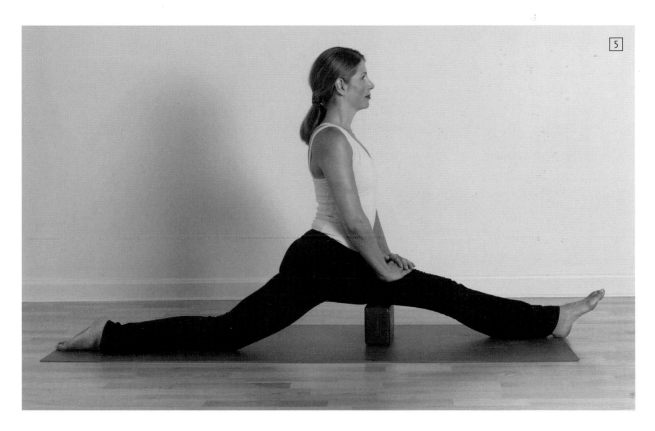

Spinal Twist Bent Leg

BENEFITS

This exercise strengthens your core in a twist. After challenging your oblique system in a twist, you will also relax in a twist after this hard-core exercise. Twists offer a variety of benefits. They help restore your spine's natural range of motion, cleanse your organs, and stimulate circulation. And they'll improve your golf swing!

1 Lie on your back, extending your heels to the ceiling, feet flexed and legs active. Slide your shoulders away from your ears, fingertips reaching long.

2 Outstretch your arms so they make a "T," palms down. Bend your knees, gluing them together. Then lower your knees to the right so they hover about an inch or two off the ground. Press the palms of your hands into the ground for trunk support and gaze at the opposite arm. Complete five full breaths, then lift your knees to the center.

3 Slowly drop your knees to the opposite side. Complete five full breaths and then pull your knees into your chest for a rest. After this exercise, just drop your knees to the floor on one side for a final spinal twist stretch, and then repeat to the opposite side. Or you can do the Spinal Twist in Chapter Four.

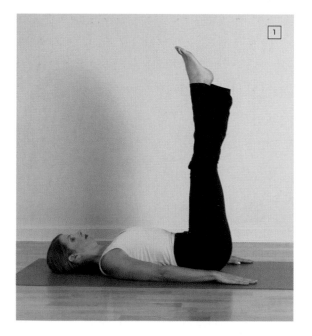

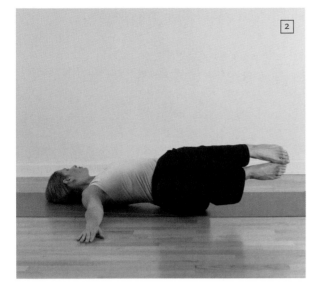

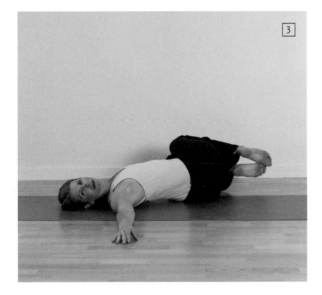

TRAINING TIPS

- If you have a spinal disc injury, then don't do any kind of twists. Please consult your doctor as well.

- If you feel any pressure in your lower back, then bend your knees or don't lower your legs to the floor. Maintain an equal balance between strengthening and good form, making sure each exhale activates the transverse for lower back protection.

- Glue your heels together, stacking them on top of one another; act as if both legs are one.

- Keep your inner thighs active and solid.

- When transitioning from side to side, make sure your bottom leg lifts the top leg to the opposite side; otherwise, you may feel tension in your lower back.

- Most importantly, elongate your spine.

- Rest in a bent knee spinal twist.

Butterfly Stretch

BENEFITS

This stretch relieves groin and lower back tension. It also calms the mind.

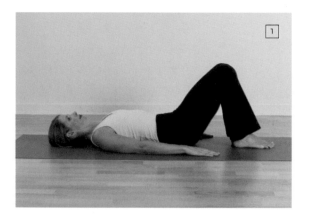

1 Lie on your back with the soles of your feet planted on the floor. Arms are by your side and relaxed.

2 Open your knees out to the side so the soles of your feet touch. Relax your hands to the side. Complete twenty to thirty peaceful breaths. You've completed the core challenge!

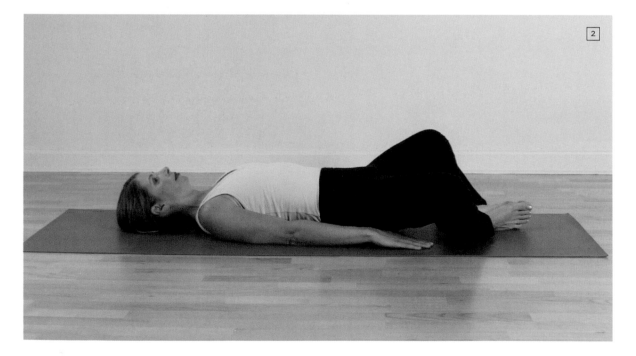

Wrapping it Up: Core Secrets

○ Given that life's movements are often unexpected, this will prepare you for the twists, slips, and falls of life. You will strengthen your body so it integrates many muscle groups in a variety of positions to challenge your body from head to toe.

○ Self-study and self-observation are vital to training. These exercises are designed to be slow and controlled so you can better listen to your thoughts and body language.

○ Lifting between your legs to activate your pelvic floor muscles assists in core stability. This contraction begins between your inner thighs, draws energy up through your groin, and ends as the contraction activates your deep abdominals.

○ The pelvic floors form the shape of a hammock where they weave through the bottom of the pelvis, from the pubic bone to the coccyx. Strengthening these muscles is good for your sex life!

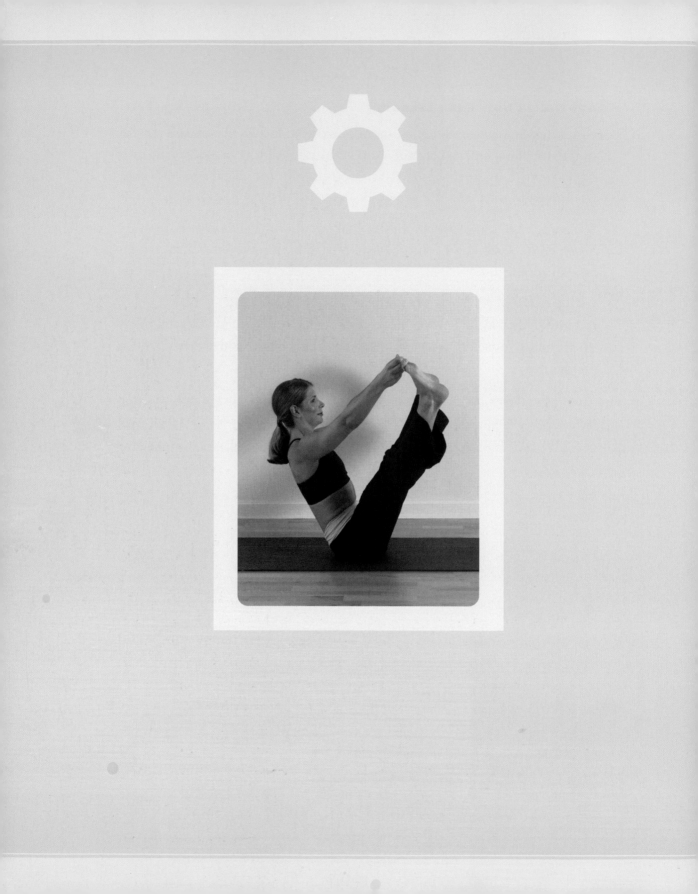

Chapter 6

Core Strength for Life

The strongest and most efficient moves spring from one thing, core strength. The next selection of exercises requires physical strength, balance, flexibility, endurance, and precision of body awareness. Mentally, you'll need tenacity, focus, courage, and solitude. This chapter is what you have been preparing for—power moves that integrate the mind, body, and core simultaneously and harmoniously. Physical strength is not enough; you must dig deep in your soul to tap into your mental fortitude. You must move consciously rather than automatically. You need to challenge yourself and not give up. These exercises are not easy. This chapter, as a whole, helps you overcome negative emotions and build self-confidence, courage, and control over your body.

How you sleep, eat, and take care of your mind are as important to your health and well-being as your physical training. Nutrition, stress management, and exercise enhance the quality of your life. Core training is one part of the whole process. There is no mind/body separation. Every move begins in the brain. As you train, challenge your mind, even when it wants to roam, to stay focused on your body while executing the exercises. As the intensity increases, the mind tells you to give up or makes up excuses why you should not try the exercise. There are frequent sips of water and the mind games—"I can't believe that I am not strong enough or good enough." Don't give in to such nonsense. There is no need to achieve perfection on every attempt, rather just try and enhance your performance each time. It's developing skills and body awareness within the movement that prepares you for life. Be present and in the moment!

BRAIN TRAINING

How does a piano player instinctively know where to place her fingers? How does a basketball player shoot from mid-air and come down in the perfect position to execute his next move? How can your body catch itself after slipping on a wet surface, never fracturing a bone? How will you train your body so it can react unconsciously in a moment of crisis? The answer is proprioception, or a certain sixth sense that involves not only the brain-to-body connection, but also the body-to-brain connection, and gives us balance. This is not just the seemingly unbelievable steadiness of a gymnast on a balance beam, but the deep-rooted kind of balance that gets you through life in one piece. This is the type of balance that most athletes possess—real-life balance! *By definition, if you possess good balance, then your body has the ability to know where it is in space.* A lack of balance can drastically increase your risk of injury. Without good balance, recovery from a fall is difficult. If you step off the curb wrong, good balance can prevent you from twisting your ankle or falling to the ground.

Like balance, good posture and core strength help you have a command over your body, which is why proprioception is often associated with core strength. Good balance also requires that many muscles, the inner ear, eyes, spine, and brain coordinate together to process the body's position. Mother Nature knew her stuff when she created us. By positioning the head directly on top of the shoulders, the shoulders over the hips and the hips over the feet, we are more stable. Muscles don't have to compensate for a perfect form, leaving your brain free to focus solely on what's happening in the body at any given moment. When you're misaligned, your brain must react to whatever situation you are in while in the midst of painstakingly trying to sort out awkward posture and distress signals from all the unhappy parts of your body. As this lag time increases with greater misalignment, suffering an injury is a very real possibility. Lack of training can also increase your risk of injury, which is why, if you practice balance movements, then you are training both your muscles and brain to react in the moment.

THE POWER OF PROPRIOCEPTION

Proprioception means a certain sixth sense that knows where the body is in space. In fact your body tells your brain where it is in relation to other objects and what's around it at all times. This is why you can perceive whether you're standing up straight or about to fall over. Improving proprioception enhances the brain-to-body connection and the body-to-brain connection. In short, balance. By definition, good balance requires that many muscles, the inner ear, eyes and brain coordinate to process the body's position in space.

HARD CORE

Here is your Hard Core workout. These exercises are for life. You can strength train with them as often as you wish:

Standing Core Activation   (Chapter Five)

Wide Leg Shoulder Stretch   (Chapter Five)

Active Hamstring Stretch (optional, Chapter Four)

Abdominal Series: Multi-Level Ab Work, Leg Wheel, Twist Curl Ups

Knees to Chest Stretch

Spinal Extension Series

Bottom Balance Series

Plank Series: Front, Side, Back

Active Child's Pose

Shoulder Stretch

Handstand Pike off the Wall

Deep Hip Flexor Stretch

Full Plank with leg extension

Full Plank with two point extension

Bonus Advance Work: Stability Ball Exercises

Abdominal Series:

Multi-Level Ab Work, Leg Wheel, Twist Curl Ups

BENEFITS

This series strengthens all of the layers of the abdominal muscles, plus tests your coordination and provides a hefty dose of core control. As the legs and arms challenge the core, keep anchoring your spine to the floor.

Multi-Level Ab Work

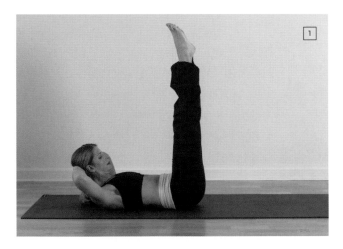

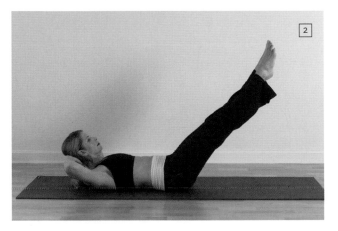

1 Lie on your back with your heels reaching toward the ceiling. Integrate your fingers and place them behind your head for support. Curl your chin to your chest to lift your shoulder blades off the floor. Anchor your spine to the floor.

2 In five steps, lower your straight legs to the floor. In the first step, lower your toes about 30 degrees. Hold here and complete five breaths.

(Multi-Level Ab Work, continued)

3 Drop down another 30 degrees so your toes are in line with your nose and exhale deeply to hug your abs to your spine. Hold for five full breaths.

4 Drop down another 30 degrees, pulling up through your inner thighs even more. Complete five full breaths.

5 Drop your heels until they hover about two inches from the ground. After five full breaths, take one more inhalation. And then exhale deeply to float your legs to the starting position. Focus on exhaling, exhaling, and exhaling to engage your core and pelvic floors to protect your lower back. Great job—this ab work series is a toughy!

TRAINING TIPS

- Hold each level for five full breaths, exhaling to hug your navel to the floor—imaging your belly button melting to your spine, as if they are one.

- Maintain a neutral stable pelvis and spine. If your low back arches or pops up from the floor, then bend your knees. And you don't have to lower your legs to the floor right away—working with good form is more important than trying to do the exercise.

- Pelvic floor contraction is crucial while you lower your legs—remember to direct energy up through the inner thighs. Pull your pubic bone to your navel and your navel in and up under your ribs, scooping a "C" in your abdomen.

- Rest by pulling your knees to your chest.

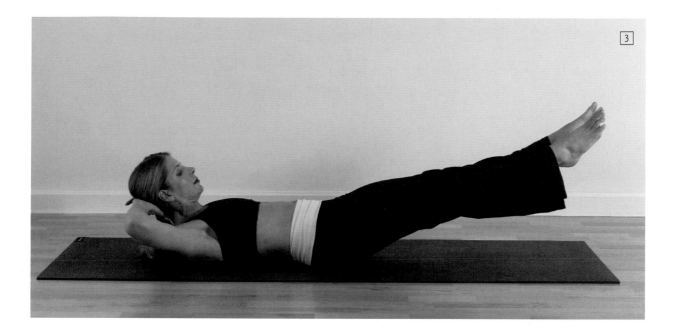

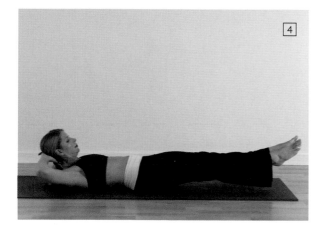

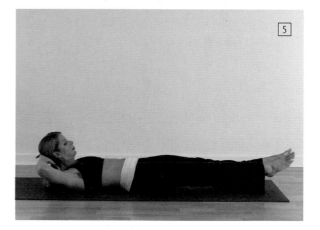

Leg Wheel

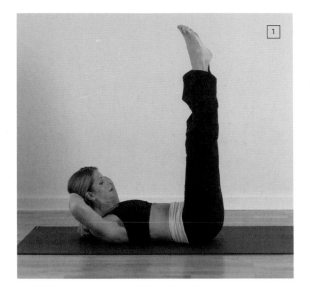

1   Lie on your back, legs straight up.

2   Inhale and then slowly lower your legs until they are about two inches from the floor.

3   Exhale as you drag your toes across the floor to the buttocks, anchoring your spine the whole time.

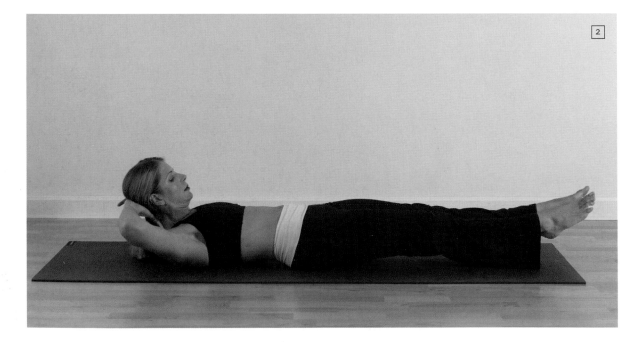

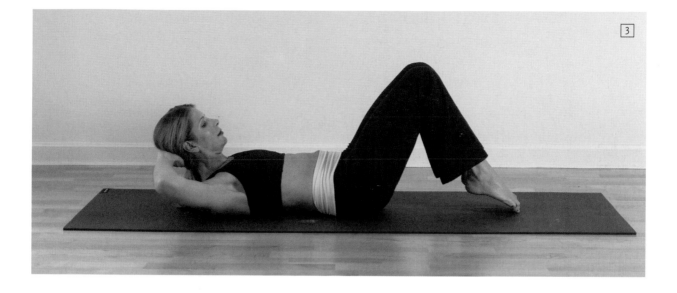

4 As you continue the exhale, lift your toes from the floor, reversing your curl by lifting the sacrum off the mat, and lengthen your toes to the ceiling. Finish in the original starting position. Begin your next inhale and complete another full circle with your legs. Complete three to five circles.

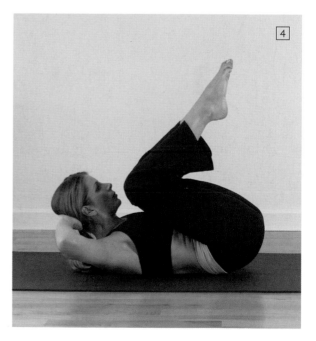

Twist Curl Ups

1 Lie on your back. Lengthen your legs out straight and extend your arms over your head, placing the palms of your hands together.

2 Inhale to prepare. In one motion, exhale and curl up, lifting your right leg to the ceiling and twisting to reach your arms past your right knee. Exhale deeply to activate all of your abdominal muscles. Inhale and stretch your arms behind you as you lay back to the starting position.

3 Exhale to curl up, lifting your left leg to the ceiling and twisting the other way. Reach your arms, with your palms of your hands glued together, past your left leg. Inhale to starting position with your arms outstretched behind you. Complete five sets, focusing on your breath each time. Pull your knees to your chest to rest.

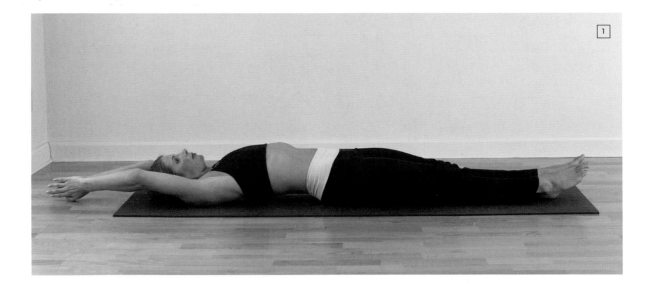

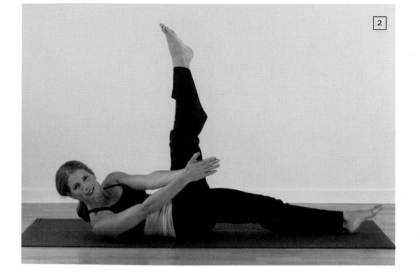

2

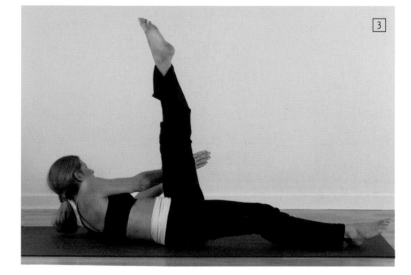

3

SELF-TALK TO VICTORY

Self-talk yourself into focus, control, and concentration to enhance your overall performance. If you can stay focused while doing these exercises, then you are working toward self-mastery. Clearly, mental training takes practice; it is not easy to master your own mind. Any time your brain is trying to talk you out of something, counter with, "Yes, I can!" That's positive self-talk along with some self-affirmation. Both are great mental training techniques that will help you work toward self-improvement.

Full Spinal Extension Series

BENEFITS

This exercise strengthens the muscles running down the back of your body and increases the flexibility of your upper back, shoulders and chest.

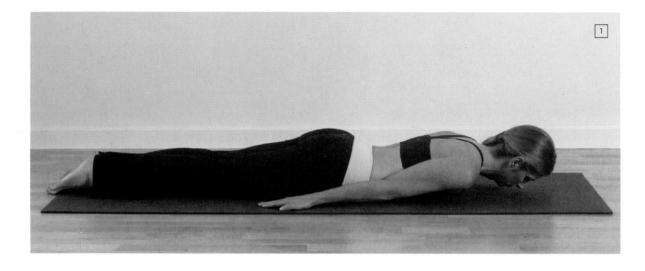

1 Lie on your stomach with your arms lengthened by your side, palms down. Your legs lengthen behind you and are open about hip-width. Rest your head comfortably on your chin and gaze at the floor.

2 Inhale to lift your arms and legs off the floor in one motion. Reach your fingertips toward your toes and interlace your fingers to help peel your chest off the floor. Send energy through your legs while lifting higher and higher. Elongate your spine from the top of your head to your toes, while resting your body weight on the pit of your abdomen. Complete five full breaths, staying in this position.

3 Still breathing into your extension, separate your fingers and reach back, palms down. (If you feel any back strain, stop and rest in an Active Child's Pose.)

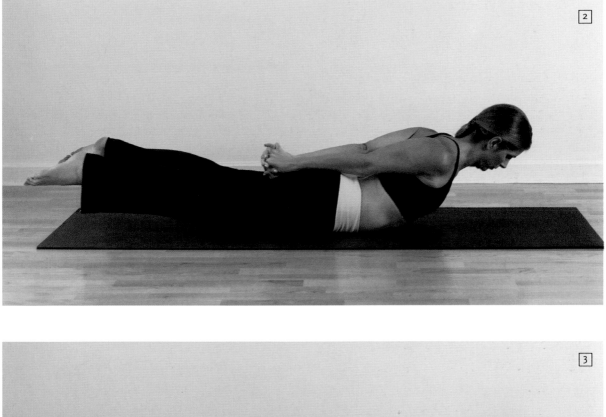

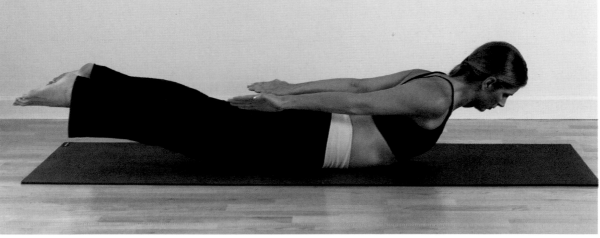

(Full Spinal Extension Series, continued)

4 Keep lifting and move your arms to make a "T" with your body. Complete five full breaths.

5 Then, reach your arms over your head for full spinal extension. Continue lifting your legs even higher to challenge your back muscles. Complete five full breaths. Stop to rest in Active Child's Pose if you need to, or keep moving through the series.

6 Next, move your arms to your waist, palms down, and try opening your legs, creating a wide "V," to challenge those hard to tone areas—your outer thighs!

TRAINING TIPS

- Don't lift your chin to the ceiling. If you shorten your neck muscles, you may experience neck strain. Rather, gaze at the floor.

- Keep lengthening through your spine, from the top of your head to your toes.

- Keep your energy moving out through your legs and arms to keep them active and solid. Balance on the pit of your belly as you lift your limbs to strengthen your back and stretch your abdominals.

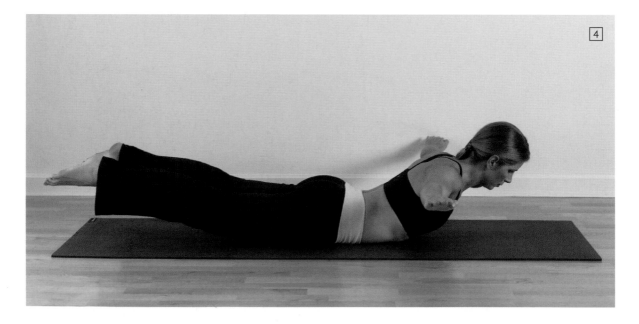

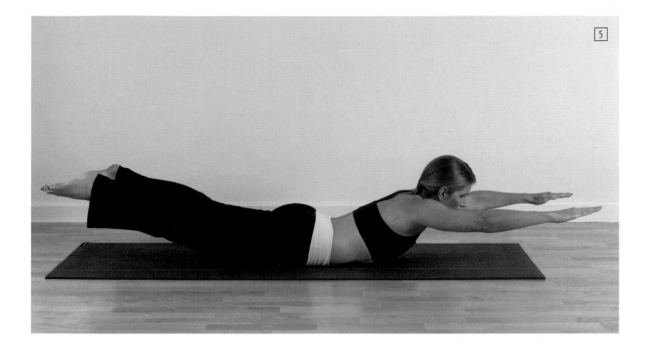

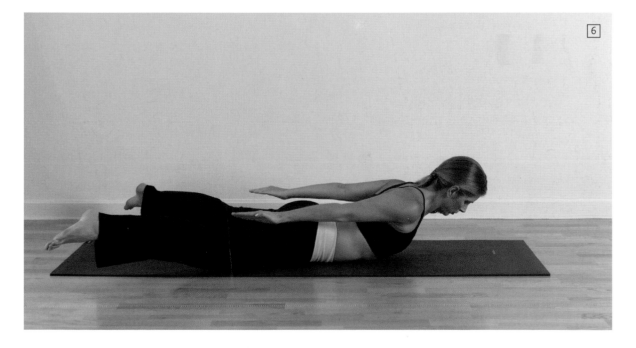

Bottom Balance Series

By honing your focus in a variety of balance positions, your levels of concentration will increase. This exercise tests your focus as you move your limbs in a variety of positions while balancing on your behind. You have two goals: the belly moves the bones of the pelvis; your breath helps stabilize your core, and calms your mind, warding off all types of distractions—keep exhaling!

1 Sit on your bottom with your knees bent and feet flat on the floor, pulling your heels in about an inch or so from your butt-bones. Place your hands on the back of your thighs. Inhale and tilt your pubic bone, scooping so deeply that you lift your toes off the floor. Stay here, exhale and regain your balance.

2 Then, in one motion, reach your fingertips and toes to the ceiling, creating a "V" with your body. Complete five full breaths.

3 Grasp your big toes with the fist two fingers of each hand, hugging your belly button toward your spine to create pelvic stability. If you need to, you can bend your knees to make your toes easier to reach, before straightening your legs back up to the ceiling. While you are in this position, challenge your core even more by opening your legs out to a "V," scooping your belly. Complete five full breaths and slowly return to the starting position. Roll onto your back to pull your knees to your chest for a stretch.

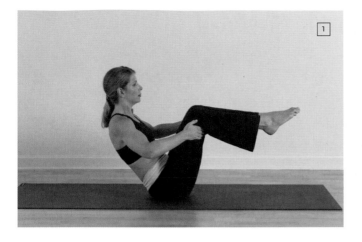

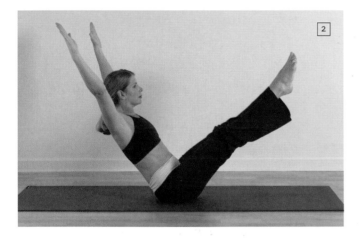

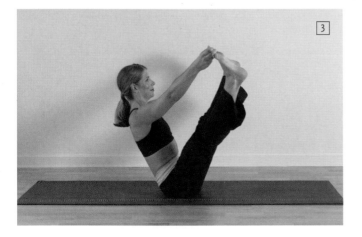

TRAINING TIPS

- If your pelvis rocks, scoop your pubic bone deeper to your navel, creating a "C." The deep abdominals move and stabilize the bones of the pelvis, so scoop, scoop, and scoop.

- When you feel unstable, your shoulders might have a tendency to creep toward your ears. Your shoulder blades are as important as your pelvis in strengthening your core, which keeps you from teetering or falling over. Remember, pits to your hips.

- If you feel any lower back pressure, first exhale to relieve the strain. If that does not work, bend your knees (look at the first picture in the steps of this exercise) until you build enough strength to extend your legs, or simply pass on this exercise.

- Don't collapse your spine or roll back on top of your tailbone. Instead, elongate from your tailbone through the top of your head.

- If you can't reach your toes, gently hold onto your calves or use a strap.

THE BENEFITS OF BALANCE

Balance exercises provide a sense of mastery over your body and promote a feeling of lightness, like you're floating. You will also gain self-confidence as you strengthen the muscular integrity of your body.

The Full Body Plank Series:

Front Plank, Side Plank, Reverse Plank

BENEFITS

This Plank series soars in intensity because your arms are straight. Planks take strength, stability, balance, and mind-control to control your body. Planks work just about every muscle in your body against gravity: abs, back, pelvis, glutes, legs, shoulders, arms, and pelvic floor muscles. This sequencing is also more challenging. You will transition from Front Plank to Side Plank in one movement and then reverse the sequence so you work the Side Plank on the other side. After completing both sides of the body, you will finish with a Reverse Plank.

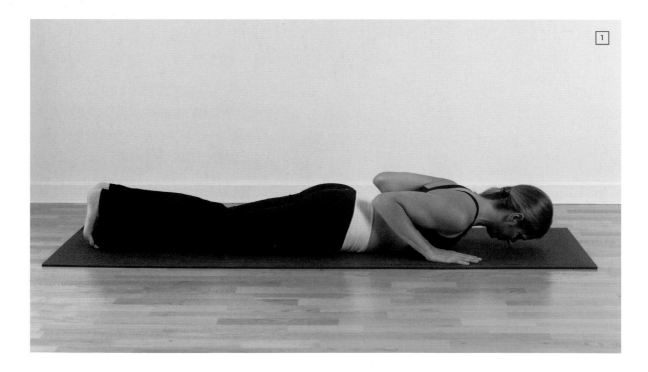

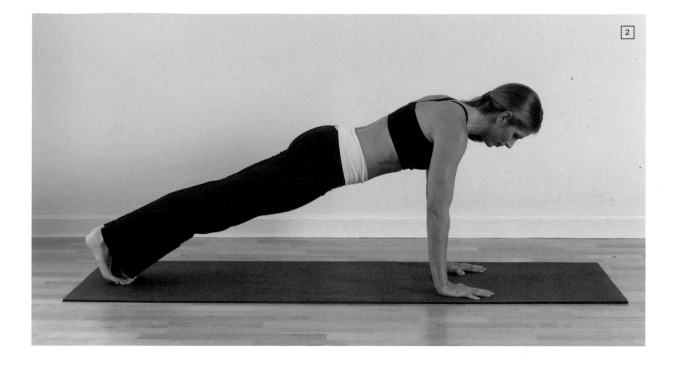

1. Lie on your stomach, face down. Place your hands directly under your shoulders, palms down. With your toes curled under, place your heels together.

2. Push up to a full plank—*remember head to heel like steel, no sagging through your center.* Complete five full breaths and then follow the directions in the next exercise to transition into a Side Plank.

TRAINING TIPS

- If you have a wrist, elbow or shoulder injury, then skip these planks.

- Maintain a solid core, strengthening your waistline. Don't sag in the center.

- Rotate the inner elbow to the front to help slide your shoulder blades down your back to create upper back stability. But don't lock your elbows.

Side Plank

<table>
<tr>
<td>1</td>
<td>

From Front Plank, rotate your body to the left so you shift your weight onto your left hand and the edge of your left foot, rotating the right side of your body into the air to point to the ceiling. *Everything between your hips and your heels should touch and stack on top of one another!* The palm of your left hand is directly under your shoulder. Your right hand rests on your upper thigh. For a final balance challenge, lift the straight arm to the ceiling. But, don't settle your body weight into your resting wrist, rather send energy up through your fingertips. Complete five full breaths and transition back to a Front Plank. Then pivot to the opposite side and complete five full breaths.

</td>
</tr>
</table>

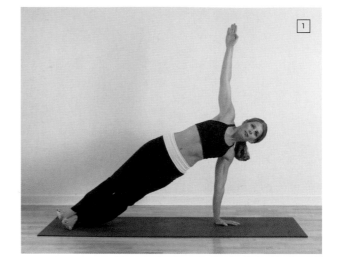

TRAINING TIPS

- Maintain a solid core, especially in the transition phase.

- Try sending energy up to the ceiling through the finger tips of your lengthened arm. This way, you can avoid putting too much pressure on your resting wrist.

- Stack your hips and heels on top of one another, channeling energy through your pelvic floor muscles.

Reverse Plank

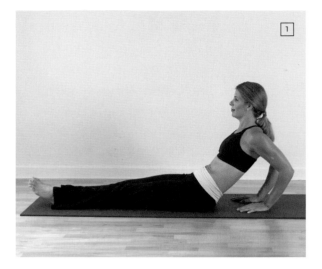

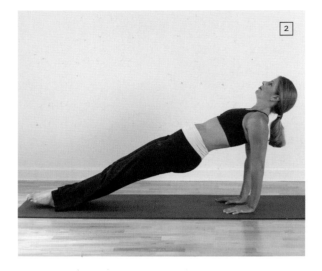

1 Sit on the floor, legs straight out in front of you. Place the palms of your hands behind you, fingertips facing your torso or out to the side. Your shoulders are directly over your hands, elbows facing back. You may feel a slight stretch across your chest.

2 In one move, lift your hips, bottom, and chest to the ceiling. Gaze at the ceiling. Point your toes to the floor to relieve any pressure you may feel in your knees. *Lift your hips higher and higher as if a sling from the ceiling hoists your hips.* Complete five full breaths and then rest in an Active Child's Pose.

TRAINING TIPS

- If you have a wrist, elbow or shoulder injury, then don't attempt planks.

- In all planks, glue the inner thighs together, engaging your pelvic floors. Feel free to use a rolled up towel in these exercises as well.

- Don't lock your elbows, yet keep your arms active— lift your energy up!

Shoulder Stretch

Now, take one more opportunity to stretch your shoulders and the front of your body.

✿ THE POWER IN AN EXHALE

Another way to relax the nervous system is to exhale deeply; it calms the mind, reduces fear, and controls your emotions—the highs and the lows. Breathing can alter most bodily functions. In fact, breathing can either calm or excite your entire nervous system. The connection between breath and emotion has long been established; it has been said "when the breath is still, so is the mind."

1 Lie on your stomach and outstretch your arms to the sides to form a "T," palms face down. Relax your legs. Take a few breaths to clear your mind; you have worked very hard up to this point.

2 Lift your left hand to the ceiling while using your legs to lift your torso from the floor.

3 Then lower your left hand behind you to connect with your opposite hand on the floor, rolling your body to open your chest away from the floor. Keep your head in a relaxed position. Try to connect your hands as gravity stretches the shoulder that rests on the floor. Complete twenty to thirty breaths, then stretch the opposite side. Finish this routine with the deep Spinal Twist and Butterfly stretches found in Chapter Five. If you want more of a challenge, then move to the super-advanced exercises.

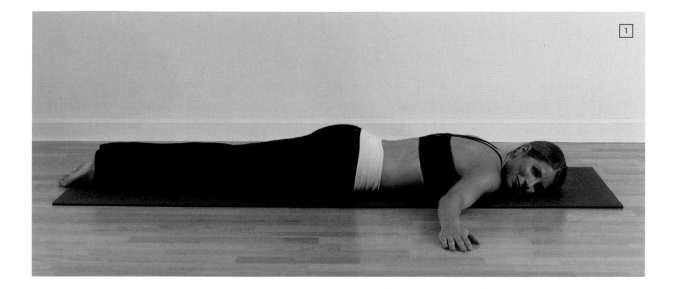

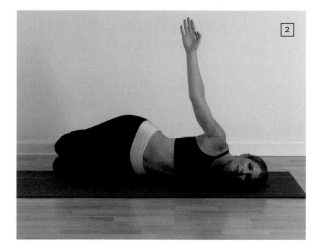 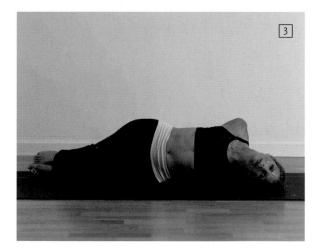

Enhanced Hard Core Exercises:

Half Handstand Pike off the Wall

BENEFITS

This exercise strengthens your core against gravity and works your body in an integrated way—gaining balance, strength, flexibility, and focus. Turning your work upside down also gives your vital organs a much needed rest and improves your circulation, respiration, and elimination. You may find yourself thinking more clearly as inversion work increases mental concentration and clarity. This exercise requires a fair amount of shoulder flexibility and mega-watts of core strength; it's challenging and spine-tingling all in one. Here's a warning: If you can't hold a Plank in good form for fifteen breaths or more, then you're not ready yet for this exercise. You might also ask yourself, "Am I willing to fall?" Because you might!

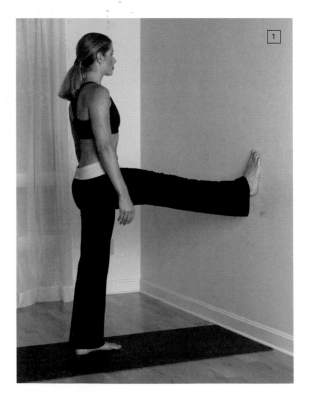

1 Face the wall and lift your leg and touch the wall with your foot to measure the distance between you and the wall. This is your starting position.

2 Turn away from the wall, but remain basically in the same place. Bend down and place your hands on both sides of your legs, by your feet. Begin to transfer your weight to your hands.

3 Walk your feet up the wall to hip height, keeping your knees tucked. Keep tucked until you feel secure on the wall. Now is the time to evaluate whether or not your arms can hold your body weight.

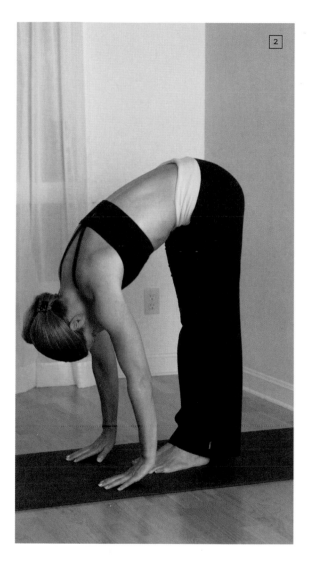

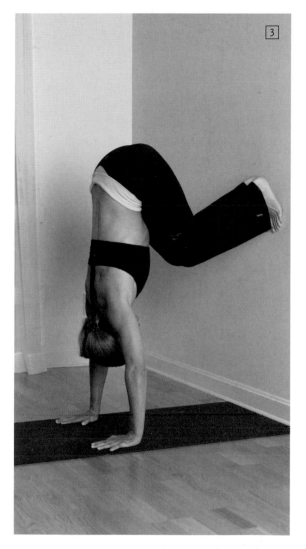

(Half Handstand Pike off the Wall, continued)

4 When ready, straighten your legs to form a ninety degree angle, or pike position with your body. Ground the soles of your feet into the wall for stability. Keep your core solid, and send energy up through your center so you don't settle your body weight in your wrists. Complete five full breaths and then walk down the wall. If you want more of a challenge then follow the next step.

5 Lift your left leg, toes reaching to the ceiling, keeping your pelvis stable. Return your leg to the pike position. Then lift the right leg. Complete three sets and then walk down the wall to get in position for the Standing Shoulder Stretch in Chapter Five.

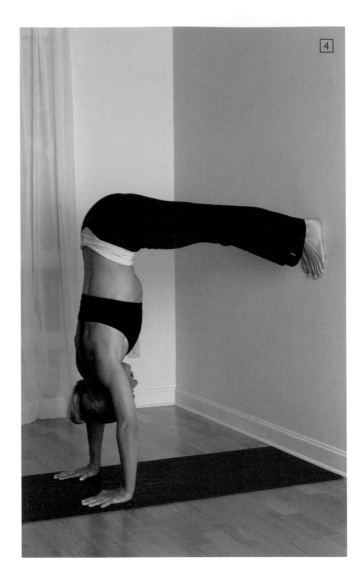

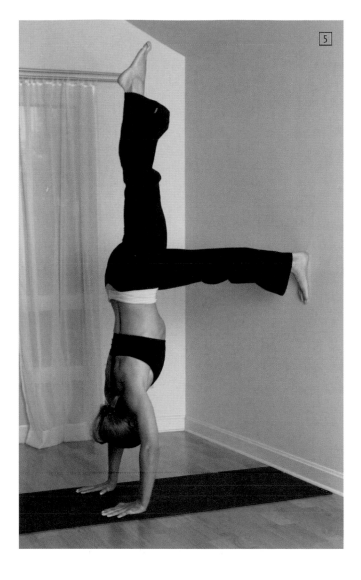

TRAINING TIPS

- The pelvis must remain stable and neutral. Don't roll your hips; this may cause you to lose your core stability.

- By lifting your legs, you are making your bottom work for its good tone.

- Your torso is directly over your arms.

- If you feel that you are collapsing in your shoulders, lift up through your arms and surge energy through your core.

- Keep the arms as straight as possible without locking your elbows.

- Engage your pelvic floors to help you from collapsing in your shoulders, wrists, and arms.

- If you have a wrist or shoulder injury, then don't do this exercise.

Deep Hip Flexor Stretch

BENEFITS

This exercise stretches your thighs and their deep muscles, such as the quadriceps and hip flexors.

1 Face the wall and lift your arm to measure the distance between you and the wall. This is your starting position.

2 Turn away from the wall, remaining basically in the same place. Bend down and place your hands on both sides of your legs, by your feet. Place your leg on the wall so your shin bone touches the wall with the top of your foot flat against the wall. Use your hands to support your body.

3 Slide your leg down the wall until you feel a deep stretch in the front of your thigh. After your knee touches the floor, use your hands for balance as you position your leg into a deep lunge. The goal is to stretch deeply enough so the thigh bone of the leg on the wall becomes parallel with the floor. Your bottom should move away from the heel of your foot to prevent you from bearing down on your kneecap. Pay attention to the alignment of the leg on the floor as well. In the deep lunge, your knee should stay directly over your heel.

4 If you have the flexibility, bring your hands to the lunging knee and stretch up through your body.

TRAINING TIPS

- If you have or had a knee injury, then pass on this stretch.

- If you feel any knee pressure, check your alignment. Your body weight should not rest directly on top of your kneecap; instead, the thigh bone should be almost parallel with the floor.

- If you don't feel comfortable stretching on the wall, then refer back to Hamstring and Psoas Stretch in Chapter Five. This stretch takes you deeper, but the stretch in Chapter Five will give you the same benefits—you must feel comfortable in your own body.

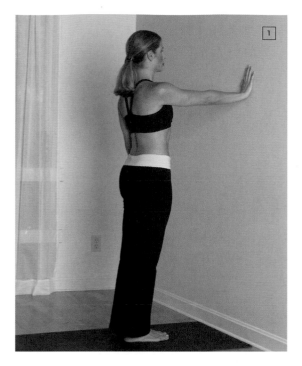

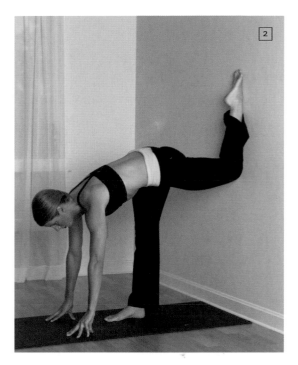

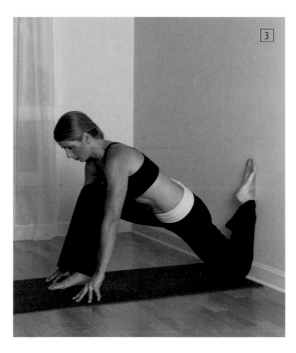

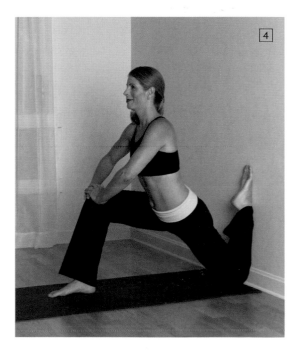

Plank with Extension Series

BENEFITS

Soon you will discover that planks are ideal for training your core muscles and just about every other muscle in the body. In these planks, you can count on maximum total body toning benefits. Here's your mantra—maximize your maximus!

1 Lie on your stomach, face down. Place your hands directly under your shoulders, palms down. With your toes curled under, place your heels together. In one motion, push up to a full plank.

2 Extend your left leg so your heel reaches toward the back wall. Your core contracts, lifting your navel to your spine, and your buttock is solid—*maximize your maximus*. Complete five breaths and then switch legs. Next, try the two point extension, which ramps up the core challenge.

3 In a full plank position, extend your right arm so your fingers lengthen away from your torso, pulling up through your core as much as possible.

4 Then lift your left leg, reaching your heel to the back wall. As you try to steady yourself, *imagine a tug-of-war between your fingertips and your toes, pulling away from one another to create a firm core.* Complete five full breaths and then switch arms and legs. Release tension in your lower back by resting in Active Child's pose.

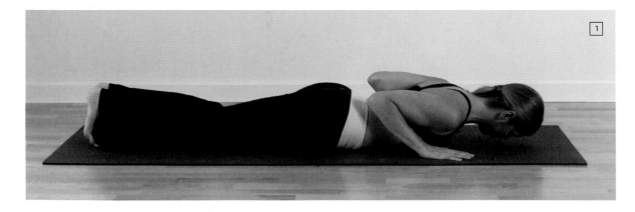

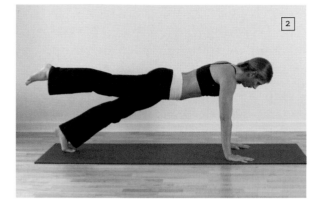

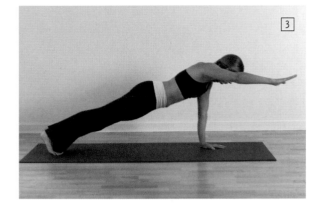

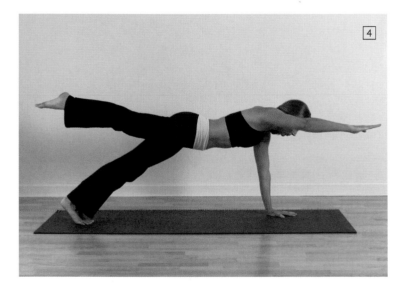

TRAINING TIPS

- If you have shoulder or a wrist injury, then don't do this exercise.

- Your fingertips must lengthen one way and your toes the other, creating a firm, taut, core—active limbs!

- Don't let your mid-section sag, which puts too much pressure on your lower back.

- Gaze at the floor.

ROLL OUT THE BALL

The stability ball is the latest craze to roll in. But how does it get your body into shape? In two words—core strength! It's a balancing act worth trying, especially if you are longing to work your torso even more, not to mention fine-tune your upper and lower body as well. These exercises roll several workouts into one. Whether you are sitting on your bottom or balancing on your toes, you are using your core to keep the ball from rolling out from underneath you. If you lose your balance, then just roll with it and have fun. Some exercises you will recognize—you have already done them. But that doesn't make them easier! Look for the intensity level written next to the exercise, so you don't end up taking a ride you did not anticipate. Below is quick exercise ball benefit review:

- ☼ The ball works the trunk in almost every exercise, plus your limbs.

- ☼ The ball improves balance, posture, body awareness, and coordination because of the dynamic nature of the ball; it rocks and rolls.

- ☼ The ball develops your strength, flexibility, and mental concentration, all rolled into one.

- ☼ The ball allows you to practice falling in a safe environment—your home. Learning to fall is a skill that you can benefit from, especially as you age.

- ☼ And finally, it's a lot of fun.

THE ULTIMATE BALANCE CHALLENGE

As you get older, the fear of falling becomes a scary possibility. Many people avoid challenging activities, further decelerating their balancing skills. Working on the ball increases the intensity of most of these exercises. This challenge is what you need to sharpen your balance skills for now and later in life. Try closing your eyes for the ultimate balance challenge. Yes, you may roll off. But is that so terrible?

SIZING TIPS

In general, when seated on the ball, your knees should be even with, or slightly above, your hips. The firmer and bigger the ball, the more difficult the exercises; the softer and smaller the ball, the less difficult. Balls generally come in three sizes: 45-cm, 55-cm, and 65-cm. Most people use the 55-cm, which is for people 5' to 5'8, and the 65-cm for taller individuals. You can buy a stability ball, sometimes called Resist-A-Ball, Swiss Ball, or Physioball, at your local sporting goods store.

Finding Neutral

BENEFIT

This exercise introduces you to balancing on the ball. And though finding neutral is relatively easy, the wobbly surface of the ball makes it a bit more challenging. Focus on reconnecting with your own inner strength and potential.

1 Sit directly on top of the ball, grounding your butt-bones. Bend your knees and plant the soles of your feet on the ground, ankles in line with your knees and feet hip-width apart. Lengthen through your spine, stacking your shoulders over your hips and ears over your shoulders. Hug your abs to your spine.

2 Tip your pubic bone to your belly and move your pelvis into an anterior tilt. The ball will roll with you, so be careful.

3 Now, move to a posterior tilt by tipping your pubic bone to the floor. Complete five full sets, making sure your belly moves the bones of your pelvis. Return to a neutral spine.

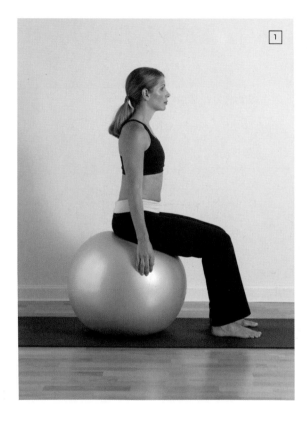

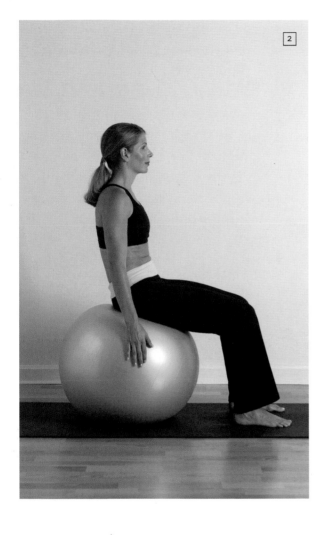

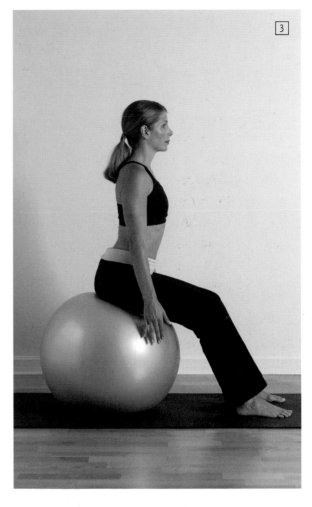

Finding Neutral with Lifted Leg

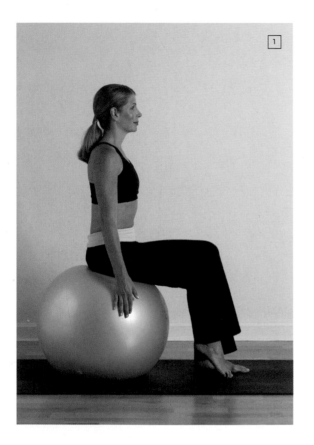

1 Sit on the ball in a neutral position, with your feet firmly grounded, about hip-width apart. Sit tall, elongating your spine and stacking your shoulders over your hips and ears over your shoulders. Hug your abs to your spine and lift one foot slightly off the floor to test the waters. Keep your butt-bones grounded evenly into the ball.

2 If you feel stable, then pull your abs to your spine and extend the right leg, without compromising your neutral spine. Complete five full breaths, return to the starting position, and then repeat the exercise with the other leg.

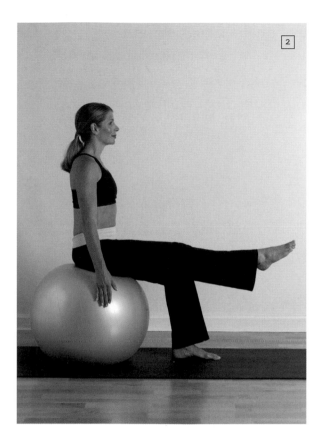

2

TRAINING TIPS

- When you extend your leg, the ball may roll out from underneath you. Focus on maintaining a neutral spine, lengthening from the spine and engaging your core to keep you steady on top of the ball.

A BALL TIP

If you are deskbound, consider sitting on an exercise ball while working. By sitting on a ball, you can strengthen your core and relieve lower back pressure, because you must sit with good posture to avoid falling off the ball. Plus, you can do those much needed mini-stretches throughout the day, so your muscles don't rebel by tensing up from sitting in one position all day.

Ab Curl Ups

BENEFITS

You may vary the degrees of intensity for strengthening your abs just by repositioning your body on the ball. The closer your bottom is to the floor, the less of a workload for your abs, making more work for your quads as they stabilize your body. The farther away your bottom is from the floor, the more work for your abs. When strengthening your abs in this position, pull your ribs to your hips and always keep your chin tucked to your chest.

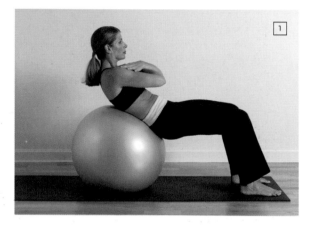

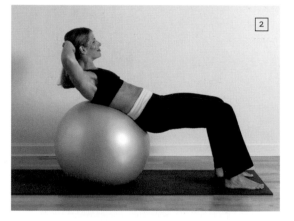

1 For beginners, sit on the ball with your feet firmly planted and slightly wider than hip-width apart to provide more stability. Lengthen from the spine and engage your abs. Walk your legs out from the ball so your lower back rests against the ball— you are basically in a seated squat position. Fold your hands across your chest. Holding this contraction may be enough of a workout for your abs!

2 To increase the intensity, walk your legs out from the ball and lift your bottom away from the floor. This time, your lower and mid back should connect with the ball while your upper back, shoulders, neck, and head are off the ball. Interlace your hands behind your head. Tuck your chin to chest and curl your torso as high as you can off the ball.

INTERMEDIATE

Ball Bridge

BENEFITS

This exercise strengthens your spine as a whole (plus hamstrings, inner thighs and buttocks), as it stretches your abdominals, quads, and hip flexors. In this ball bridge, you will begin by sitting in neutral. Keep in mind that your foot placement makes the exercise more challenging. If your feet are slightly wider than hip-width, you will have more stability. If, on the other hand, you tighten up the distance between your feet, then the exercise becomes more difficult. If you want the ultimate challenge, then lift one leg.

1 Sit on the ball with your feet firmly planted and slightly wider than hip-width apart to provide more stability. Lengthen from your spine and engage your abs. Walk your legs out from the ball so your upper back rests against the ball—you are now in a table top position. Rest the back of your neck on the ball and cross your arms across your chest. Lift your hips to the sky. Complete five full breaths and then return to the starting position.

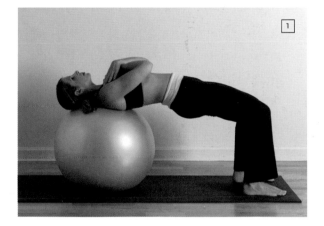

TRAINING TIPS

- For proper alignment in this ball bridge, make sure that your head is in a comfortable position resting on the ball. Don't hang your neck off the ball.

Spinal Extension: Bending Over the Ball

BENEFITS

Now let's curl your spine the opposite way. Since most abdominal exercises curl forward or curl up, you need to counterbalance that work with extension. You have learned in previous chapters that the extensor muscles of the back work in harmony with the abdominals, creating a strong core. Not only will extension on the ball strengthen your back muscles, but your legs and arms as well. The goal in this series is similar to what you have already learned, but since extension is crucial to the development of a healthy spine, here are a few tips. The goal is to keep your core active while your legs and arms work; elongate slowly through the spine—no need to rush. Don't lift your chin to the ceiling, which puts needless pressure on your neck; instead, keep your head in line with your spine.

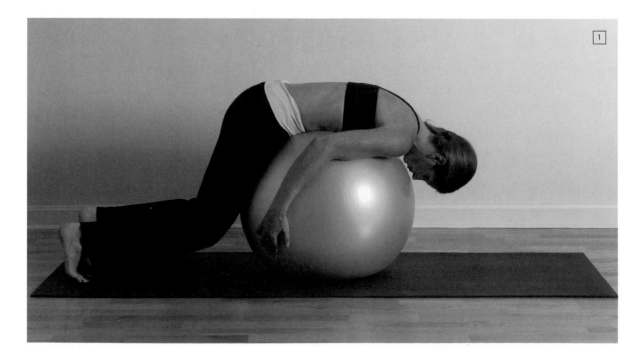

1

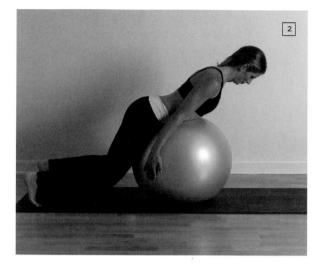 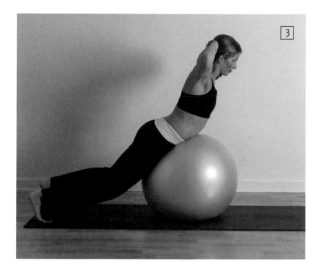

1. In a kneeling position, drape your body over the ball while holding the ball steady with both hands. Your knees are slightly bent and your toes are tucked, providing a little extra stability.

2. With your hands holding onto the ball, lift your chest off the ball; elongate from the base of your spine to the top of your head. Complete five full breaths and then relax in the starting position. Beginners, stop here.

3. Follow the same starting position instructions and then, when you are ready, interlace your fingers and place them behind your head. Then lift your whole torso off the ball, lengthening from the base of your spine to the top of your head. Complete five full breathes and return to the relaxing position.

(Spinal Extension, continued)

4 To advance the extension, begin the same way. However, in this extension, lift your straight arms to the ceiling—fingertips lengthen as the spine stretches. Complete five full breaths and then relax in the starting position.

5 For a resting ball move, just drape your entire body over the ball.

TRAINING TIPS

- The idea is to elongate and stretch the spine. Don't over-arch your back.

- Slide the shoulder blades down your upper back.

- You may bend your knees. If you want to increase the intensity of this exercise, straighten the back of your legs.

- Lengthen the back of your neck—head in line with spine the whole time.

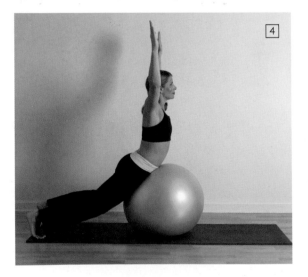

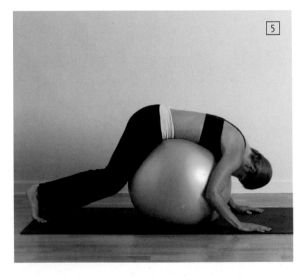

INTERMEDIATE TO SUPER-ADVANCED

Plank to Pike

BENEFITS

In these planks, the entire body will be strengthened as a unit—not just your core, but your arms and shoulders, plus your hips and legs. Depending on your ball skill level, you have a few choices as far as increasing the intensity. To make planks easier, anchor your pelvis on the ball; for intermediate work, anchor your knees on the ball and, for advanced, the ball will end up near your shins or ankles. With your legs resting on the ball, your core will suspend in mid-air, so you must hug your abdominals to your spine at all times.

1 To get in position, kneel in front of the ball and drape your torso over it. Walk your hands until you are in a plank position, pelvis resting on the ball. Ground the palms of your hand into the floor and extend your feet out behind you. Your wrists are in line with your shoulders, and your head lengthens. Your elbows may be slightly bent, but not locked. Complete five full breaths and then roll the ball underneath you to bring you to a resting position.

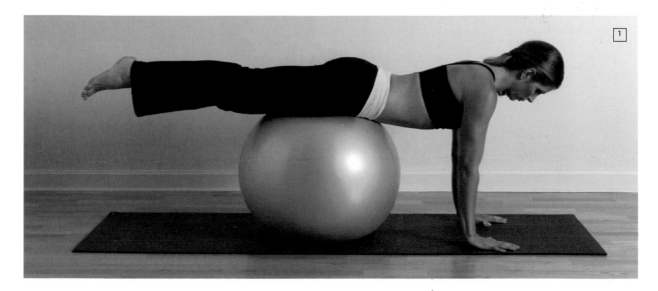

2 For an intermediate plank, walk your hands out so your knees rest on the ball. Complete five full breaths and then roll the ball underneath you to come to a resting position.

3 For an advanced plank, walk your hands out so your ankles or shins rest on the ball. Even though you have some support from the ball, keep pulling up through your pelvic floors. This plank is extremely difficult, so you need to focus on the core as a unit—don't droop in your center. Complete five full breaths and then roll the ball underneath you to bring you to a resting position.

4 For a super-advanced plank, try extending your leg. Begin in the advanced plank position where the ball is at your ankles, walking your hands out so your wrists are directly under your shoulders. Pull your abs to your spine and lift one leg. Hold the leg extension for five full breaths and return to the plank position so you can repeat the extension on the opposite leg. Drape your body over the ball for a soothing spine stretch. If you want more of a challenge, then try Pike.

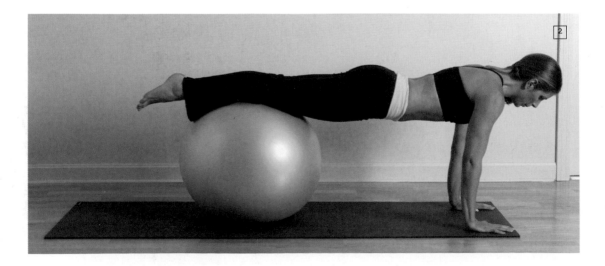

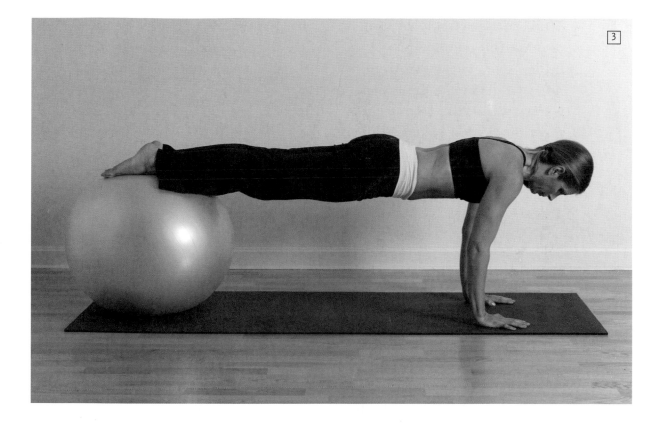

3

TRAINING TIPS

- To alleviate wrist pressure, consider using a pair of dumbbell weights. Hold the weights so your wrists don't bend at the joint, and maintain a neutral position.

- You must hug your abs to your spine the whole time. If you can't keep the ball steady, try exhaling deeper and deeper to activate your core.

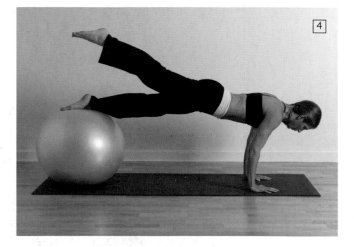

4

(Plank to Pike, continued)

5 After Leg Extension Plank, you must cool off your lower back before attempting a Pike. There is no real technique to this stretch, the best way is to kneel in front of the ball and crawl on top, walking your hands out for support. Drop your head, and relax. Think of this stretch as an Active Child's Pose on the ball.

6 Get in the same starting position in a plank with the ball at your ankles. Walk your hands out to an advanced plank, legs straight and active. Your wrists are in line with your shoulders, your elbows are secure, but not locked. Take a breath to focus on the movement and then, as you exhale, lift your hips to the sky, contracting your abdominals to the max. Complete five full breaths, exhaling deeply to position your hips over your shoulders, and shoulders over your wrists. Relax by stretching the spine in a Child's Pose on the ball.

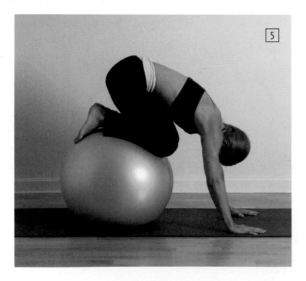

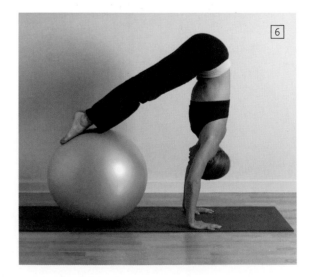

ADVANCED

Shoulder Bridge

BENEFITS

In addition to strengthening the abdominals, this exercise will work the back of your legs, bottom and hamstrings.

1 Lie on your back with your legs resting over the ball. Your arms reach alongside your thighs, fingers away from your ears to slide your shoulder blades down your back.

2 When ready, roll the ball out with your legs until they are straight, channeling energy through your inner thighs, as if your legs were one leg. Then, in one movement, lift your hips to the sky, lengthening your fingertips away from your ears to create stability. Your shoulders are stable and are in line with your toes. Complete five full breaths and then roll the ball underneath your knees to rest.

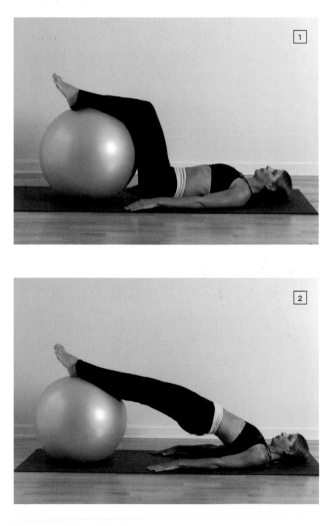

(Shoulder Bridge, continued)

3 To advance the shoulder bridge, from the first bridge position, lift one leg so your toes lengthen to the ceiling. Even as you lift the leg, pull up through your inner thighs, keeping your leg active. Compete five full breaths and then return to the shoulder bridge. When ready, lift the opposite leg.

4 To advance the shoulder bridge and strengthen your hamstrings at the same time, get in a shoulder bridge. Lift one leg to the ceiling—stabilize here. Then inhale to move the leg resting on the ball toward your bottom—engaging your hamstrings and glutes—and exhale to roll the ball way from your bottom. Try three to five sets and then switch legs.

5 After you have completed whatever level was appropriate for your skill, de-stress on the ball to release your lower back. There is no specific technique, just arch over the ball, breathe and think of the wonderful thing your just did for your body!

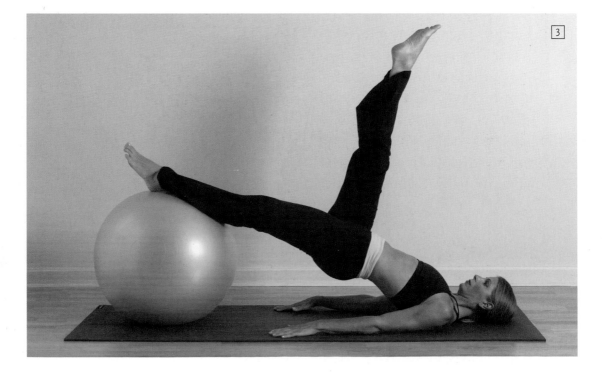

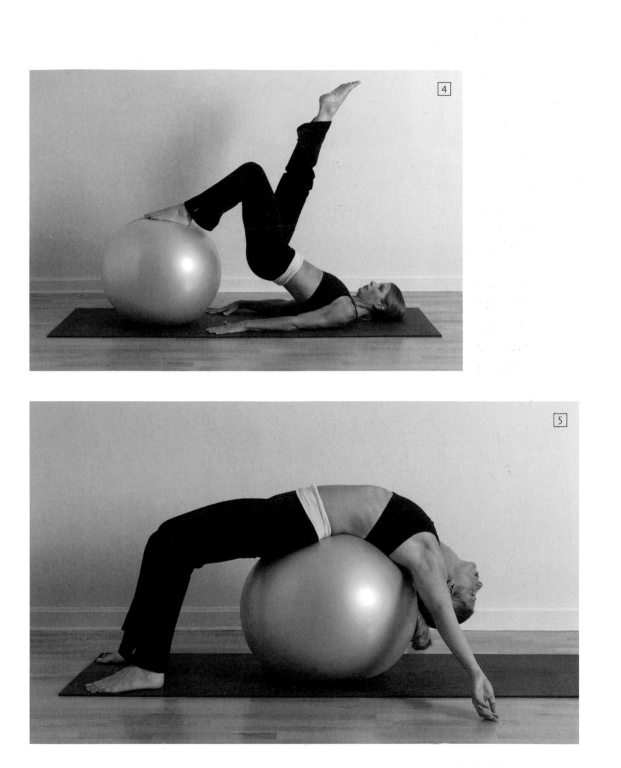

Wrapping it Up: Core Secrets

○ Brain Training engages proprioception, that certain sixth sense that improves not only the brain to body connection, but also the body to brain connection. You will train your brain.

○ By definition, good balance requires that many muscles, especially those of the core, the inner ear, eyes, and brain coordinate to process the body's position in space.

○ A lack of balance can drastically increase your risk of injury.

○ These exercises will provide you with a sense of mastery over your body, a feeling of self-confidence as you strengthen and improve the muscular integrity of your body and a feeling of lightness—as if you are floating in mid-air.

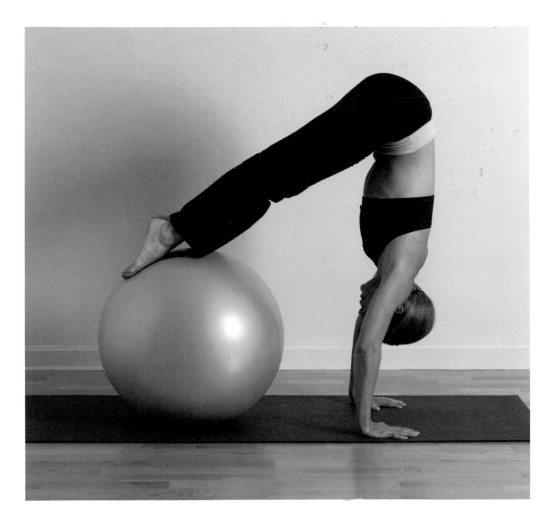

ACKNOWLEDGMENTS

When I arrived at Boston's Logan International airport, I didn't know what to expect. My mind was racing on all the work I had to do to finish my book—and then I saw my name. Wayne, my driver, greeted me with a Texas-size "Hello" and a bright smile, making me feel right at home. As we drove to Gloucester, he offered tidbits and facts about his hometown like a new father praising his baby. And, I'll never forget his words. He said, "Two wonderful things have happened to me in my life. First, I was born in the United States, and second, I was born in Gloucester." He was right on!

Thank you so much to Fair Winds Press (a division of Rockport Publishers) for such a wonderful time in Gloucester. I'm just so grateful to you for hunting me down and asking me to write this book. A special thank you must go to Ken Fund and Holly Schmidt for your hospitality—and for trusting me to deliver such a book. Of course, I'm also indebted to all you guys, including Dalyn Miller, for showing me how to eat steamers—a skill I'm sure will come in handy someday. Thank you, Paula Munier and Janelle Randazza, for entertaining me with diva-stories—I still laugh today. And thank you, Kristna Evans, for editing my manuscript with such attention to detail—you're a great copy editor. And though the photo shoot was hard work, I had a wonderful experience that I'll always remember. You're a first class art director, Silke Braun! And Bobbie Bush, you made me feel so vogue—a big Texas hug to you and your assistants. I'm also grateful that Deborah Coull and Lesley Griffin from the Deborah Coull Salon and Aveda Concept and Sanctuary Salon did my hair and makeup—I only wish I could take them home with me for daily makeovers. Kudos to *YogAndU* for providing such stunning outfits for the photo shoot. And finally, to my editor, Donna Raskin:

I'm humbled to work and learn from you and words can't describe how thrilled I am that you know fitness!

On the home front, I am so appreciative that I have wonderful people supporting me and my career. My mother is my rock. Regardless of what's happening in my life, she stands tall behind me. I love you, Mom, with all of my heart!

To my father and stepmother, I feel your love and support despite living so far away. And every girl needs a Bo! Bo Mikolajczyk, thank you for being my best friend, for dropping whatever you're doing to help me, and your kind words of encouragement, even when life doesn't work as planned. And, Kjehl Rasmussen, my hearts goes to you! I'm so lucky that you walked into my Pilates class, and especially blessed that you guided me down that precipitous legal path—and for all the hugs and emotional support. I'm indebted to Janet Harris (my writing coach) for catching my mistakes when I'm too spent to look at my own prose. I would not have a writing career if you weren't for you! And I wouldn't have core strength if I hadn't learned from such fabulous instructors such as Karen Sanzo, Colleen Glenn, and all of the other instructors who have taught me so much—I'm truly blessed! To all of my students, thank you for coming to class and inspiring me to be the best instructor possible.

And finally, thank you to my four-legged love, Kubera. I'm so happy that when you need attention, you come to me, which forces me to take a much needed stretch break. I also love that you keep my feet warm while I write—you're my best companion.

Also Available from Fair Winds Press

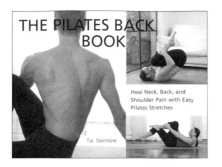

The Pilates Back Book
Heal Neck, Back, and Shoulder Pain
with Easy Pilates Stretches
By Tia Stanmore
ISBN: 1-931412-89-8
$17.95
Paperback; 128 pages
Available wherever books are sold

Most of us will experience back pain at some point in our lives, often as a result of injury or poor posture. By building inner muscular strength and flexibility, this Pilates-based exercise program gives real and lasting benefits for people suffering from backache, a sore neck or strained muscles. It can prevent you from experiencing injuries and postural problems and help you recover more quickly if you do.

The exercises are easy to follow whether you are familiar with Pilates or a newcomer. If you need to concentrate on a specific area of your back, the Upper Torso and the Lumbo-pelvic programs will guide you through the exercises most beneficial to you. This expert step-by-step program will:

• build inner muscle strength and flexibility

• reduce your risk of injuries and posture problems

• speed recovery from backaches, sore necks, and strained muscles

Tia Stanmore is a member of the Pilates Foundation and is a Pilates instructor at The Third Space in London. She has presented numerous conferences and training sessions on the use of Pilates in Physiotherapy. She is a Board Member for Dance UK Physiotherapy Advisory Board and has developed a role in injury prevention and in skill training for dancers.

Also Available from Fair Winds Press

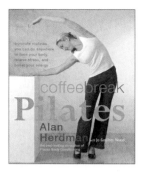

Coffee Break Pilates
5-Minute Routines You Can Do Anywhere to Tone Your Body, Relieve Stress, and Boost Your Energy
By Alan Herdman with Jo Godfrey Wood
ISBN: 1-931412-28-6
$16.95
Paperback; 144 pages
Available wherever books are sold

Whether you are eating breakfast, sitting in front of your computer, or taking the subway—whatever your age or fitness level, Pilates is the answer! All you need is 5-minutes from your busy day to improve energy and muscle tone while you center your mind and refocus. With this simple exercise plan you can do Pilates any time, any place. Getting fit has never been easier, or more convenient! This "thinking exercise" lets your body and mind work in harmony, improving your posture, calming your mind, and relieving aches and pains. Wherever you are, whatever you are doing, you can fit these exercises into your day. *Coffee Break Pilates* is the perfect equipment-free workout for a stronger, leaner, fitter body.

• Use the spare moments in your day to get fit

• Improve your posture and relieve your sore neck and strained muscles

• Easy step-by-step instructions

• No need for expensive equipment or a gym membership

Alan Herdman is an internationally respected authority on Pilates. He has worked intensively with and was trained by Pilates teachers in New York. He has since established Pilates exercise studios in several countries, including his own in London. Currently Alan's clients include artists from film, TV, theater, opera, and ballet.

Also Available from Fair Winds Press

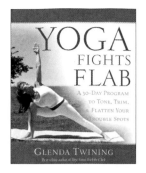

Yoga Fights Flab
A 30-Day Program to Tone, Trim, and Flatten Your Trouble Spots
By Glenda Twining
ISBN: 1-59233-058-4
$19.95
Paperback; 192 pages
Available wherever books are sold

Yoga can help you lose weight and tone up! This easy four-week program features calorie burning and muscle-strengthening to help you burn fat and create strong, sexy muscles.

Routines include:

• A 15-minute high-energy calorie burner

• A 5-minute lift-your-butt toner

• Arm and shoulder strengtheners

• A short ab flattener

Glenda Twining is a yoga instructor, fitness expert, and the author of *Yoga Turns Back the Clock*. A fitness specialist by Cooper Institute of Aerobics Research, Glenda lives and works in Dallas, Texas.

Also Available from Fair Winds Press

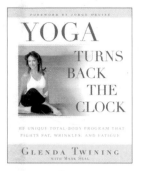

Yoga Turns Back the Clock
The Unique Total-Body Program that Fights Fat, Wrinkles, and Fatigue

By Glenda Twining
ISBN: 1-59233-006-1
$19.95
Paperback; 192 pages
Available wherever books are sold

> "This yoga book stands out from the crowd. Straightforward and no-nonsense, the rejuvenation-yoga connection is noteworthy and inspiring."
> —Ann Louise Gittleman, author of *The Fat Flush Plan*

There is a magic formula for staying young—yoga!

You can be as toned, energized, and beautiful as you were in your twenties—or more so! Yoga practitioners have long known the secrets to looking and feeling young. Now you can harness the amazing power of this ancient art to fight flab and rejuvenate every part of your body with the three energizing routines in this book.

Through simple step-by-step instructions and easy to follow full-color photos, Glenda Twining shows you the miracle of anti-aging yoga. She has helped hundreds of people turn back the clock with her unique program, and you can be next!

You'll learn:

• Why 30 minutes is all it takes to transform your body

• How yoga works to rejuvenate your entire body from the inside out

• Simple stretches you can do at home to fight fat and feel younger

Glenda Twining is a yoga instructor, fitness expert, and author of *Yoga Fights Flab*. Certified as a fitness specialist by the Cooper Institute for Aerobics Research, she lives and works in Dallas, Texas.